X-Ray Interpretation for MRCP

Charles R. K. Hind

BSc (Hons) MD MRCP
Consultant Physician in General and Respiratory Medicine
Royal Liverpool University Hospital
and The Cardiothoracic Centre, Liverpool

SECOND EDITION

D0682133

CHURCHILL LIVINGSTONE
EDINBURGH LONDON MADRID MELBOURNE NEW YORK AND TOKYO 1992

CHURCHILL LIVINGSTONE
Medical Division of Pearson Professional Ltd

Distributed in the United States of America by Churchill
Livingstone Inc., 650 Avenue of the Americas, New York,
N.Y. 10011, and by associated companies, branches and
representatives throughout the world.

First edition 1983 (Pitman Publishing Ltd)
   Reprinted 1986 (Churchill Livingstone)
Second edition 1992
   Reprinted 1993
   Reprinted 1994
   Reprinted 1995

ISBN 0-443-04551-8

British Library Cataloguing in Publication Data
A catalogue record for this book is available from the
British Library.

Library of Congress Cataloging in Publication Data
Hind, Charles R. K. (Charles Robert Keith)
    X-ray interpretation for MRCP/Charles R. K. Hind.-
    2nd ed   p.   cm.
    Includes bibliographical references and index.
    ISBN 0-443-04551-8
    1. Diagnosis, Radioscopic-Examinations, questions, etc.
  I. Title.
    [DNLM: 1. Radiography-examination questions.
    WN 18 H662x]
RC78.15.H56 1992
516.07′572′076-dc20
DNLM/DLC
for Library of Congress   91-23535
                                                CIP

The
publisher's
policy is to use
**paper manufactured
from sustainable forests**

Produced by Longman Singapore Publishers (Pte) Ltd
Printed in Singapore

Preface to the second edition

In the eight years since the first edition of this book, there have been changes in the written part of the MRCP (part II) examination.

Firstly the slide projection of X-rays has been abolished. Now each candidate is given a booklet containing prints of each radiograph together with the question, and writes his/her answer adjacent to each print.

Secondly, there is an increasing trend in recent years to include more clinical information in the stem of each question. This is for several reasons, not least of which is to test the candidate's ability to make more sensible suggestions in the light of the clinical details.

Thirdly, the range of radiographic material has been extended to include computed tomography of the chest and abdominal ultrasonography.

Finally, of course, there are new medical conditions (e.g. HIV infection, AIDS) which not only have their own particular radiographic features, but also have to be included in the differential diagnosis of certain X-ray abnormalities.

The second edition of this very popular book reflects these changes in examination content. Though the total number of questions remains the same, I have included more CT scans and added in some ultrasound pictures. Furthermore several of the original X-rays have been replaced by better quality prints. For the use of these new X-rays I am indebted to my radiologist wife, Fiona Fraser, and to Dr Austin Carty of the X-ray Department at the Royal Liverpool University Hospital.

Otherwise the purpose of the book remains the same — to help you pass the MRCP (part II) examination. Good luck!

Liverpool, 1991   C. R. K. H.

Preface to the first edition

The idea of writing this book arose originally from the wide range of interesting radiographic material I encountered whilst a Registrar in General Medicine at Ealing Hospital, and latterly from my experience in teaching MRCP candidates at the Hammersmith Hospital. I am indebted to Dr Ann Heller, Radiologist at Ealing Hospital, for providing the vast majority of the X-rays reproduced here, and for her help and enthusiasm during the book's production. Additional material is reproduced by kind permission of Professor R Steiner and the staff of the X-ray Department at the Hammersmith Hospital, Professor D K Peters and Dr R Eban.

I would also like to thank Ms Katharine Watts of Pitman Books; Fox and Waterman, photographic developers and printers; and Ms Denise Brinkman for her characteristically excellent secretarial assistance.

London, 1983   C. R. K. H.

Contents

Introduction

The examination for the Membership of the Royal College of Physicians' diploma (MRCP) includes compulsory questions on photographic prints of X-rays. This is not intended to be a specialist examination, but designed to select those suitable for higher training in general medicine and its related specialties. Its aim is to test clinical competence and knowledge. Some candidates fail because they do not have these qualities. Many more fail because of inadequate preparation for the examination, and/or lack of technique. The aim of this small book is to correct both these sets of faults when interpreting X-rays. Both photographs and questions are designed so that candidates will become familiar with the type of X-rays shown, and the extent of the radiographic knowledge required in the MRCP (part II) examination. Candidates may also practise their technique, both in interpreting the X-rays, and in answering accurately the types of questions set.

In part II of the MRCP examination, the photographic print section consists of 20 compulsory questions, each based on a print or pair of prints. On average, one-third of these are of X-rays. The question should be read carefully, as it often contains a clue to help with interpretation of the X-ray. Every candidate should have a practised and thorough system for looking at each type of X-ray likely to be encountered. The abnormalities shown are often straightforward, in the middle of the print and seen immediately. In many cases, however, the changes are either multiple, or not immediately seen. It is then only by applying a systematic approach to each film that one or all of the abnormalities will be seen. When one abnormality has been identified, the candidate should look again at the rest of the film, both in general for other abnormalities, and specifically for changes that may be associated with the one already noted. For example, the most likely cause of a hilar mass in a middle-aged smoker is bronchogenic carcinoma. Other radiographic features should be specifically looked for; for example bony metastases, pleural effusion, or evidence of phrenic nerve involvement.

Each part of the question should be answered accurately, and always in the light of the information provided. For example, bilateral hilar lymphadenopathy in a young West Indian woman, with a history of painful shins, is far more likely to be due to sarcoidosis than to Hodgkin's disease. Most questions have a preferred answer, which receives maximum marks. Alternative answers receive a lower mark according to a set scale, but never a negative mark. Sensible guesses are therefore worth while. The candidate should never panic if unable to answer a few of the questions. All questions carry equal marks. If one proves difficult, time allowed for the succeeding question should not be sacrificed. Only when the next question has been confidently and completely answered, should time be spent on any previous unanswered ones.

There are five sections in the book, each containing 20 questions. It is hoped that these will be used as mock examinations. Some questions and X-rays are slightly more difficult than those set in the MRCP examination. Answers are given at the end of each section, with relevant interpretations and discussions, and details of similar X-ray abnormalities that candidates should be familiar with. In such a small book, the information contained cannot be uniform or comprehensive. If unfamiliar with any of the X-ray features referred to, candidates should look in one of the standard radiology textbooks listed in the bibliography section.

Section 1

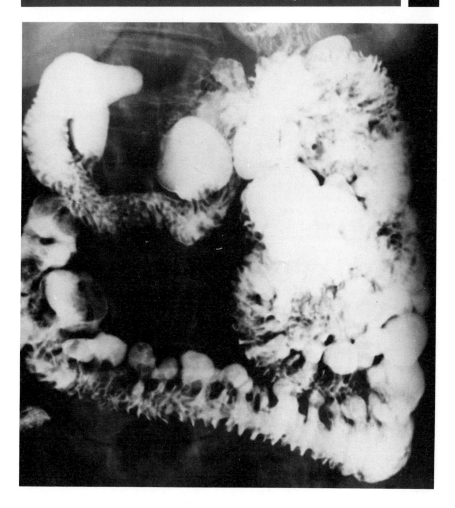

1.1

What is the cause of this lady's malabsorption?

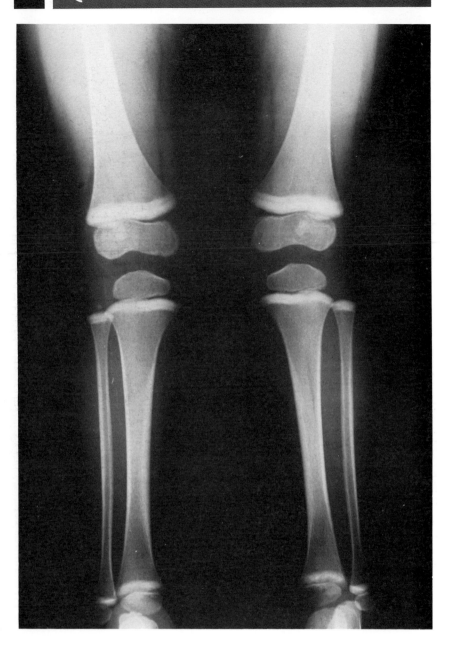

1.2

These X-rays are of a child who gives a history of abdominal pain.

a. What abnormality is shown?
b. What is the most probable diagnosis?
c. What other radiological abnormality may be found?

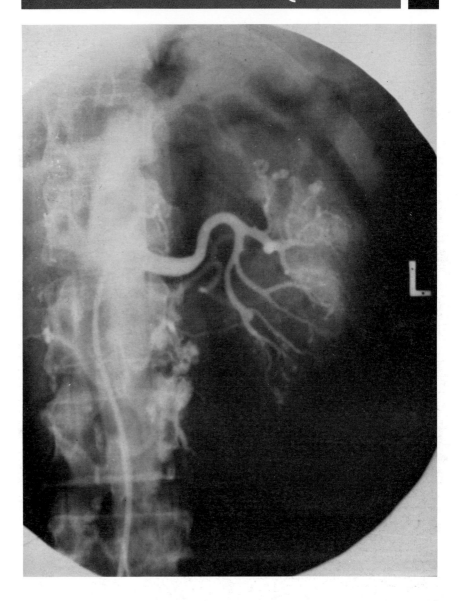

1.3

This is the renal arteriogram of a 40-year-old man with uncontrolled hypertension.

What is the most likely diagnosis?

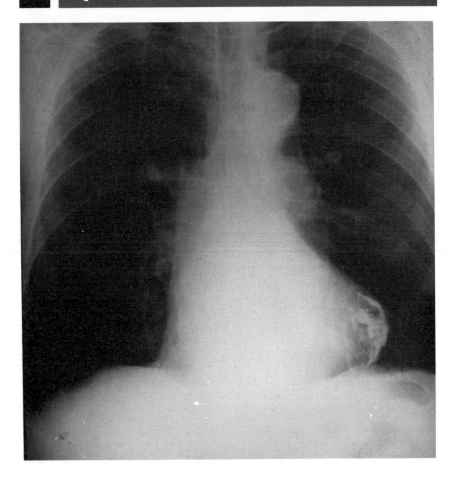

1.4

This 60-year-old man presented with heart failure.

a. Describe two abnormalities that are visible.
b. What is the most likely diagnosis?

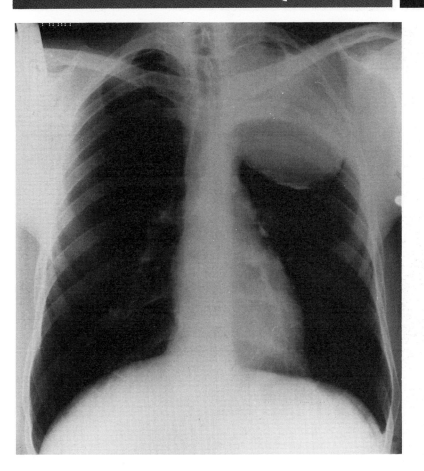

1.5

What is the cause of the abnormality shown?

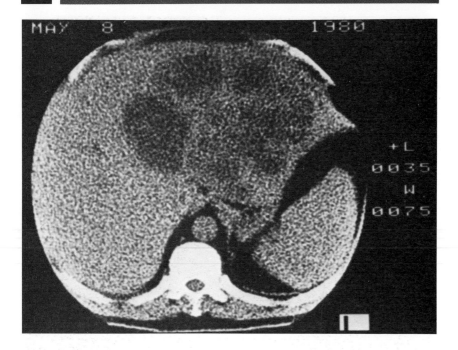

1.6

This 60-year-old man has acute diverticulitis.

What complication has arisen?

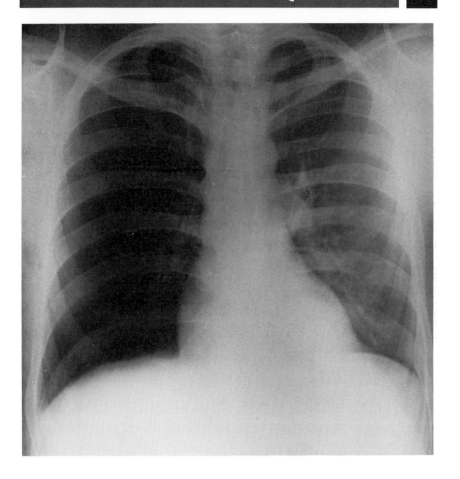

1.7

This is the chest X-ray of a 45-year-old man, taken during a routine medical examination.

a. Describe two abnormalities.
b. Suggest a possible diagnosis.

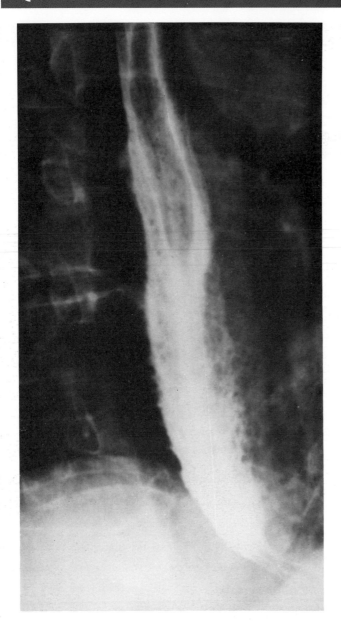

1.8

This elderly lady complained of painful dysphagia.

What is the diagnosis?

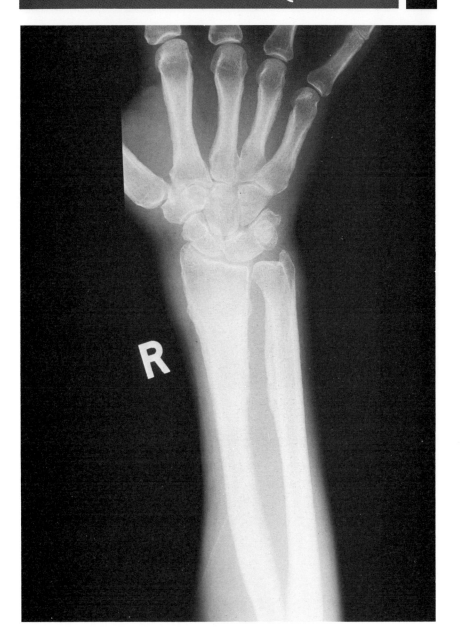

1.9

a. What is the cause of the abnormality visible on this X-ray?
b. Name three diseases with which this condition is associated.

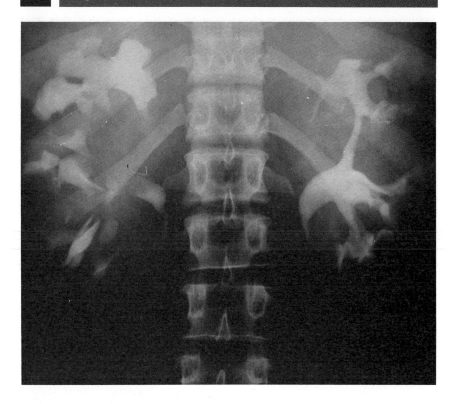

1.10
What is the diagnosis?

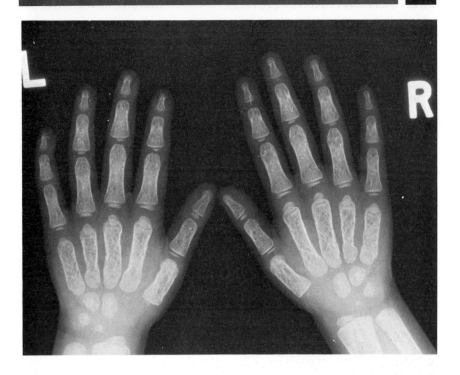

1.11

These hand X-rays are of an anaemic Italian boy.

a. What is the diagnosis?
b. What is the cause of the changes shown?

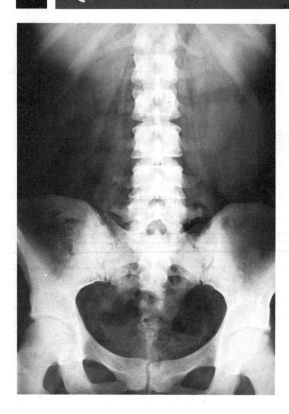 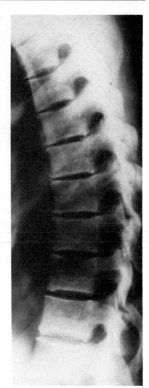

1.12

This 50-year-old man is anaemic.

a. What two abnormalities are visible?
b. What is the diagnosis?

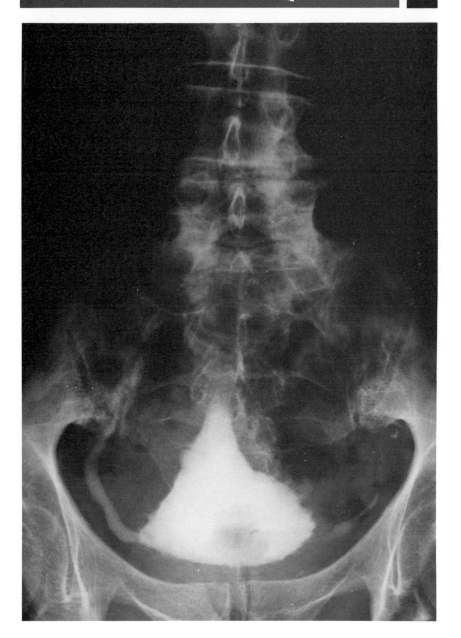

1.13

a. Describe two urological abnormalities.

b. What are the causes of these abnormalities?

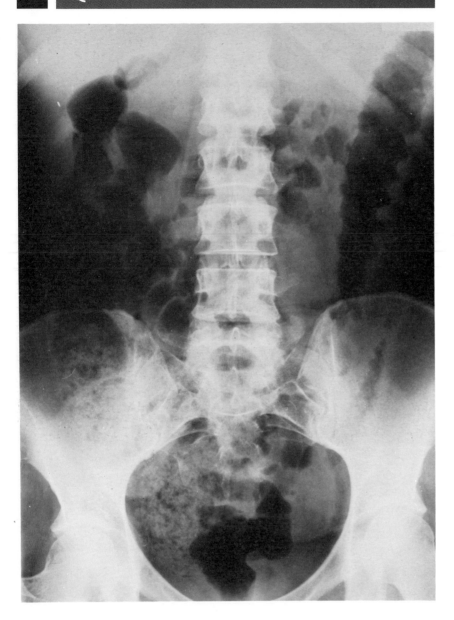

1.14

What is the most likely diagnosis?

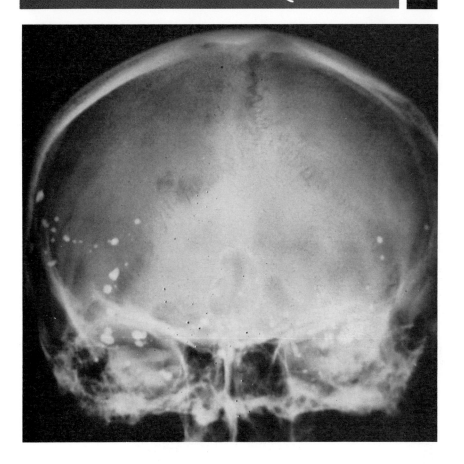

1.15

This is the skull X-ray of a 40-year-old woman who presented to the casualty department following a minor head injury.

What is the most likely cause of the abnormality shown?

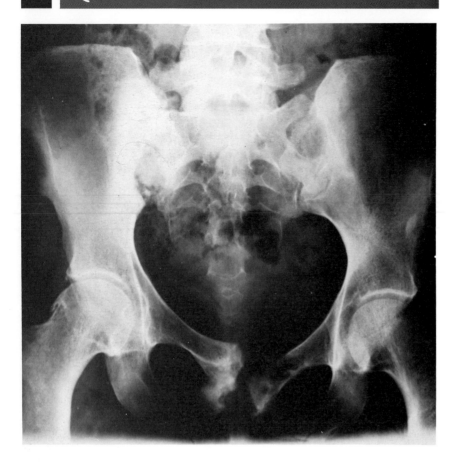

1.16

This young Indian girl presented with low back pain.

a. What two abnormalities are visible on this X-ray?
b. What is the most likely diagnosis?

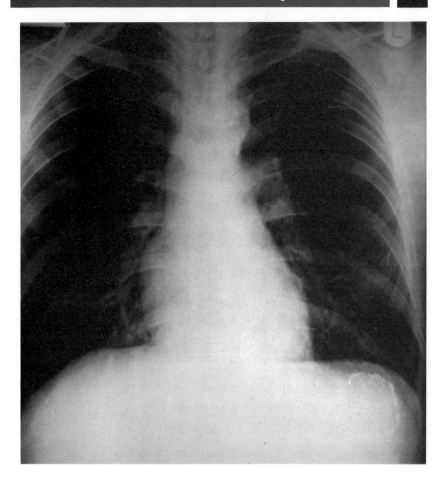

1.17

This Indian man was seen in casualty shortly after a fall.

What are the causes of the two abnormalities visible on his X-ray?

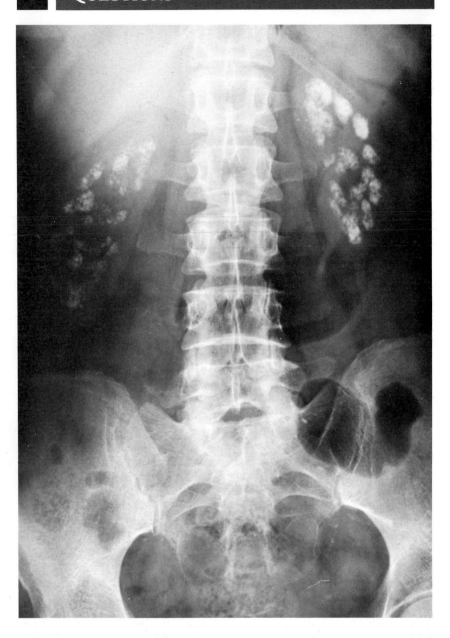

1.18

Give three causes of this radiological abnormality.

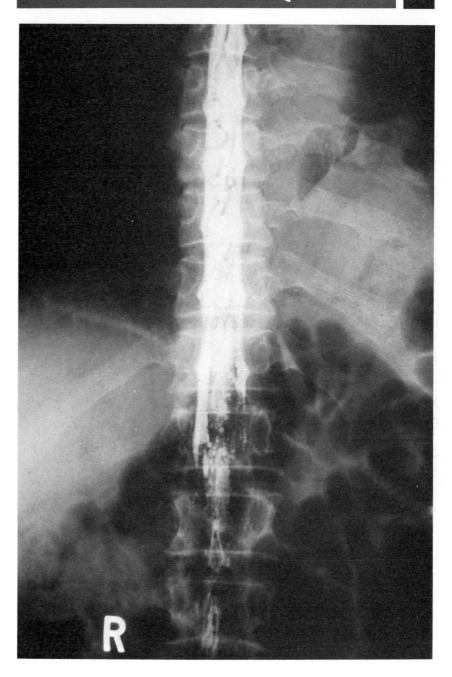

1.19

What is the cause of the abnormality shown on this myelogram?

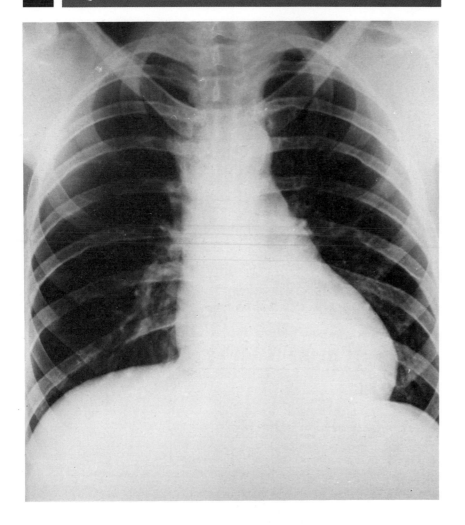

1.20

a. *What two abnormalities are visible?*

b. *What is the cause of these changes?*

1.1

Jejunal diverticulosis, with presumed bacterial overgrowth.

There are numerous smooth-walled outpouchings or sacs on the mesenteric side of the jejunal wall. Mucosal folds can be seen entering the diverticula. From a radiological point of view, malabsorption syndromes can be divided into two main groups:

1. Conditions with only the radiological features of malabsorption: namely, small bowel dilatation (normal jejunal diameter is less than 26 mm; ileal 23 mm), thickened mucosal folds, and flocculation of the barium (this feature is dependent on the type of contrast medium used). Such non-specific signs are seen in:
   a. Diffuse lesions of the intestinal mucosa: coeliac disease, tropical sprue, Whipple's disease.
   b. Deficiency of absorptive factors: enzymes, pancreatic juice or bile.
2. Conditions with specific radiological features:
   a. Localized lesions of the small intestine: Crohn's disease, lymphoma, scleroderma.
   b. Anatomical lesions: bowel resection, jejunal diverticulosis, blind loops, fistula.

Figure 1.1a shows the normal feathery pattern of concentrated barium in the small intestine.

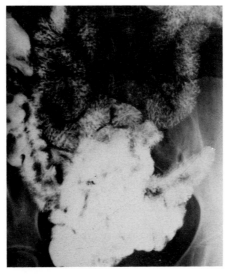

Fig. 1.1a
Normal barium follow-through

1.2

a. *Wide, abnormally dense metaphyseal lines.*
b. *Lead poisoning.*
c.   (i)   *Transverse bands of increased density in the diaphyses (residues from previous episodes of ingestion).*
     (ii) *Multiple dense flakes within the intestine (lead-containing paint).*
     (iii) *Changes of raised intracranial pressure (encephalopathy) on the skull X-ray.*

Lead poisoning is found mainly in children who ingest flakes of lead-containing paint from old woodwork (pica). Lead replaces calcium at the sites of greatest growth potential in the growing skeleton. The increased density is due in part to the lead itself, but mainly to the osteoblastic response it provokes. Clinical features include abdominal pain, anaemia, failure to thrive and encephalopathy. The differential diagnosis of the radiological features include:

1. Normal metaphyseal density.
2. Healed rickets.
3. Fluorosis: chronic ingestion of water high in fluorine in endemic areas (Persian Gulf, India, China) leads to more generalized sclerotic changes (Fig. 1.2a).
4. Other heavy metal poisoning: of historical interest only:
   a. Bismuth: used in the treatment of syphilis between 1920 and 1943.
   b. Phosphorus: now in the heads of safety matches (rarely causes sclerosis).
   c. Radium: scientific workers only at risk.

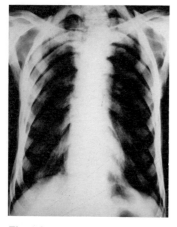

Fig. 1.2a
Fluorosis: generalized
osteosclerosis, with more
diagnostic irregularity of the
lower ribs

1.3

Classical polyarteritis nodosa.

There are multiple intrarenal aneurysms, a finding in 60% of these cases. In addition, there are less specific signs of arteritis, with variation in vessel calibre and 'cutting-off' of some vessels (found in 25% of cases). These findings in either the renal or hepatic circulation were thought pathognomonic of classical polyarteritis. However, similar findings have now been reported in a few cases of systemic lupus erythematosus. In polyarteritis nodosa, hypertension is found in 70% of cases, and is more common among those in whom intrarenal aneurysms are demonstrated at angiography.

1.4

a. (i) *Localized bulge of the left lower cardiac margin.*
(ii) *Calcified area at the apex.*
b. *Calcified left ventricular aneurysm.*

Such calcification may arise in a thrombus overlying an area of infarcted myocardium without frank aneurysmal formation. In calcific pericarditis, calcification is not normally seen at the apex on the postero-anterior film. It usually overlies the atrioventricular grooves and right ventricle, appearing as a linear plaque on the postero-anterior film, and as a thick arc or circle of calcification on the lateral film (Fig. 1.4a).

Other causes of cardiac calcification are:

1. Calcification of the left atrium, in chronic rheumatic heart disease. Usually along the postero-superior aspect, as straight or curved lines a few millimetres thick.
2. Calcification of cardiac valves: mitral or aortic most commonly. In congenital, degenerative or rheumatic valve disease.
3. Atheromatous coronary arteries, or a coronary artery aneurysm (Fig. 1.4b).
4. Calcified patent ductus arteriosus (Fig. 1.4c).
5. Calcified intracardiac tumours: myxoma, metastases.
6. Calcification within the great vessels: aorta (atheroma, syphilis) or pulmonary trunk (pulmonary hypertension).

A localized bulge of the left lower cardiac border is also seen with primary or secondary tumours arising in the myocardium. In Fallot's tetralogy, the bulge is usually of the upper left cardiac border, with the apex raised above the diaphragm.

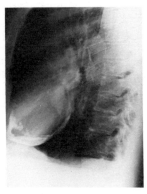

Fig. 1.4a
Calcific pericarditis

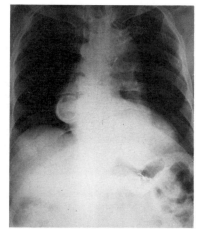

Fig. 1.4b
Calcified coronary artery
aneurysm

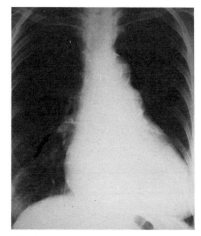

Fig. 1.4c
Calcified patent ductus
arteriosus, with left ventricular
enlargement

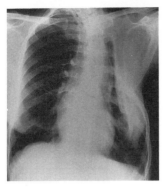

Fig. 1.5a
Left-sided thoracoplasty

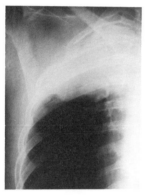

Fig. 1.5b
Pancoast tumour: destruction of
the first two ribs

1.5

Plombage.

Before the advent of antituberculous chemotherapy, 'collapse' therapy of affected portions of the lung was extensively practised. The lung was kept deflated either by thoracoplasty (Fig. 1.5a), phrenic nerve crush or by stripping off the parietal pleura from the upper chest wall to allow the apex of the lung to collapse. The extrapleural space was then either repeatedly filled by air, or packed with inert material (plombage). This was either solid (as in this case), or consisted of hollow balls (lucite, or 'ping-pong'). The subsequent radiological appearance is quite characteristic. There is an opaque area at the apex of the lung, with a smooth well-defined margin, convex downwards and medially. The overlying ribs are irregular, from previous stripping during the plombage operation. There is also evidence of previous tuberculous infection at the left hilum (irregular calcification).

The most important differential diagnosis is an apical bronchogenic carcinoma (Pancoast or superior sulcus tumour). These usually have an irregular lower margin, with a less distinct demarcation from normal lung tissue. In addition there is usually evidence of destruction of one or more of the upper three ribs (Fig. 1.5b). The extent of chest wall invasion can be more accurately assessed by CT scanning (Fig. 1.5c).

An *Aspergillus* mycetoma is usually easily distinguished. These balls of fungus originate from mycelium growing around the walls of old cavities (e.g. tuberculous), which then fall off and lie loose within the cavity. This gives rise to the characteristic radiological appearance (Figs 1.5d and 1.5e) of an opaque mass surrounded by a meniscus of air. Rarely, a similar appearance is seen with old blood clot in a cavity, or in a degenerating neoplasm.

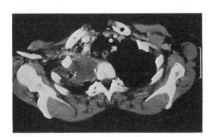

Fig. 1.5c
Enhanced CT scan: left apical
bronchogenic carcinoma
extending through the margin of
the chest wall

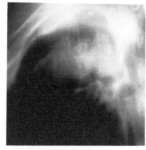

Fig. 1.5d
Mycetoma

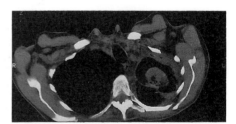

Fig. 1.5e
Unenhanced CT scan: left apical
mycetoma in an old tuberculous
cavity

1.6

Multiple abscesses in the liver.

These are numerous well-demarcated areas of low attenuation within the liver parenchyma. Radiologically, these cannot be distinguished from secondary neoplasms. In hydatid disease the low attenuation areas usually have a more defined border, and contain septae (Fig. 1.6a).

Pyogenic liver abscesses may arise in one of several ways:

1. Via the portal vein: appendicitis, diverticulitis, amoebiasis, infected colonic carcinoma.
2. Along the bile ducts: common bile duct obstruction (stone, stricture).
3. Via the hepatic artery: septicaemia.
4. Along the umbilical vein: in the newborn.
5. By direct extension: subphrenic abscess.

Ultrasonography is particularly useful in distinguishing simple liver cysts from abscesses or metastases. Cysts tend to have well-defined, thin walls and are anechoic with distal acoustic enhancement (bright signals behind the cyst — Fig. 1.6b). In contrast, abscesses tend to be thicker-walled and are usually echo-poor. Metastases are of varying size and have mixed echogenicity (Fig. 1.6c).

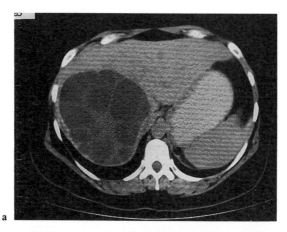

a

Fig. 1.6a
Unenhanced CT scan: hydatid disease of the liver

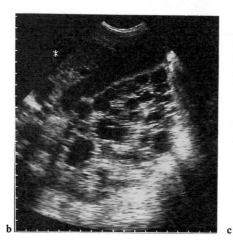

b

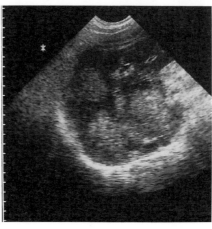

c

Fig. 1.6b
Abdominal ultrasound: polycystic kidneys

Fig. 1.6c
Abdominal ultrasound showing hepatic metastases

1.7

a. (i) *Hypertranslucent right hemithorax.*
   (ii) *Smaller right pulmonary artery with a decrease in both the size and calibre of the peripheral lung markings.*
b. *Macleod's syndrome (unilateral emphysema and arterial hypoplasia).*

This disorder follows childhood obstructive bronchitis, the resulting damage causing impaired development of blood supply, bronchi and alveoli. There are a number of other causes of unilateral hypertranslucency:

1. Changes in the chest wall (normal pulmonary arteries): mastectomy, congenital absence of pectoralis major, muscle wasting (e.g. polio), or scoliosis.
2. Pulmonary causes: unilateral obstructive emphysema (mediastinum displaced to the other side); compensatory emphysema (collapse or lobectomy); bullae (thin-walled cysts); congenital absence or hypoplasia of a main pulmonary artery (may be isolated, or part of a Fallot's: diagnosed by arteriography).
3. Pleural causes: pneumothorax; or contralateral increase in lung markings (effusion on a supine film; pleural thickening).
4. Slight rotation of the patient (commonest).

1.8

Oesophageal moniliasis.

There is an irregular ('shaggy') oesophageal mucosal outline due to ulceration. This complication may occur in patients who are debilitated or are infected with the human immunodeficiency virus (HIV), or who have been treated with antibiotics (as in this case), immunosuppressive agents or steroid inhalers.

It is usually easily distinguished from oesophageal varices (Fig. 1.8a), which appear as nodular, worm-like filling defects.

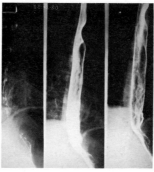

Fig. 1.8a
Oesophageal varices

1.9

a. *Hypertrophic pulmonary osteoarthropathy.*
b.   *(i) Bronchogenic carcinoma (90%): squamous cell or adenocarcinoma. Rare in oat cell carcinomas.*
     (ii) Mesothelioma.
     (iii) Rare causes: congenital heart disease, intrathoracic sepsis, pulmonary metastases from osteogenic sarcoma.

There is an exuberant periosteal reaction, with parallel amellar new bone formation ('candle-wax') along the diaphyses of the radius and ulna, and also of the metacarpals (less marked). Clinically this condition is nearly always preceded by clubbing. It causes a painful, symmetrical arthropathy similar to rheumatoid disease. Gynaecomastia, facial flushing, or excessive sweating of the hands and feet may be additional features.

1.10

Polycystic disease of the kidneys.

Both kidneys are enlarged. There is displacement, elongation and deformity of the calyces ('spider leg' appearance) by adjacent cysts. In addition, some cysts protrude into the renal pelvis, producing rounded filling defects.

     Other causes of large kidneys (greater than the length of three vertebral bodies and their discs) include renal vein thrombosis and renal infiltration (amyloid, lymphoma).

1.11

a. *Thalassaemia major.*
b. *Pronounced marrow hyperplasia.*

Marrow hyperplasia destroys the majority of the medullary trabeculae, and thins the overlying cortex of the expanded metacarpal and phalangeal shafts. Compensatory hypertrophy of the remaining trabeculae results in a coarsened pattern. Similar changes may be found in the feet, long bones and ribs. Characteristic changes may be seen on the skull X-ray (Fig. 1.11a).

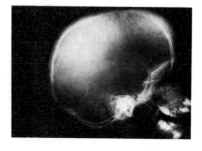

Fig. 1.11a
Thalassaemia: replacement of the outer table of the skull with perpendicular striations ('hair on end')

1.12

a. (i) *Diffuse and widespread increase in bone density.*
    (ii) *Massive splenomegaly: well-defined mass in left upper quadrant.*
b. *Myelosclerosis (myelofibrosis)*
    In splenomegaly the splenic flexure is usually depressed downwards, the left diaphragm raised and the stomach pushed forward and medially. Other causes of splenomegaly in which it may be possible to make the diagnosis radiologically are trauma (fractured lower ribs, loss of clear outline of enlarged spleen) and hydatid disease (calcified mass within the spleen).

Other causes of generalized osteosclerosis are osteopetrosis (Albers-Schönberg or marble bone disease), fluorosis (Fig. 1.2a), Paget's disease, secondary deposits (prostatic or breast carcinoma; Hodgkins' disease) and vitamin A poisoning.

1.13

a. (i) *Rounded filling defect within the bladder.*
    (ii) *Trabeculated, conical or 'pine tree' shaped bladder.*
b. (i) *Bladder catheter balloon.*
    (ii) *Neurogenic bladder.*

This may complicate congenital myelodysplasias, disseminated sclerosis, spinal cord trauma, tabes dorsalis and diabetes mellitus. Filling defects within the bladder may also be produced by bladder stones or tumour, prostatic enlargement and ureteroceles.

1.14
Active ulcerative colitis of the distal transverse and descending colon.

The extent of the formed faecal residue on the plain film gives some guide as to the proximal extent of active disease. This is confirmed in this case by an 'instant' barium enema examination (Fig. 1.14a). The distal colon is narrowed, and has a continuous, symmetrical, coarsely granular mucosal lining, with loss of the normal haustral pattern.

In contrast, the radiological features in Crohn's disease of the colon are discontinuous ('skip lesions'). Strictures and fistulae may also be seen. Ischaemic colitis results in larger, more asymmetrical 'thumbprint' deformities in the mucosa (Fig. 1.14b). Toxic dilation of the colon (where the diameter exceeds 6.5 cm) may be seen in ulcerative colitis, Crohn's disease and ischaemic colitis, and also in amoebiasis and chronic bacillary dysentery.

In long-standing ulcerative pancolitis (Fig. 1.14c), the colon has a shortened, featureless, tubular appearance, with reflux of barium through a patulous ileocaecal valve.

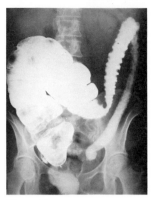
Fig. 1.14a
Ulcerative colitis

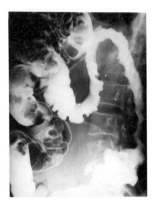
Fig. 1.14b
Ischaemic colitis: 'thumbprint' deformities due to intramural haemorrhage and oedema

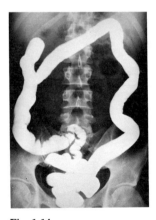
Fig. 1.14c
Total chronic ulcerative colitis: 'hosepipe' colon

1.15

Previous myodil myelogram.

There are numerous small pockets of oily myodil in the intracranial sub-arachnoid cisterns, residue of a previous myelogram. Water-soluble compounds (metrizamide) are absorbed within 24 hours, and excreted in the urine.

1.16

a. (i) *Right sacro-iliitis.*
    (ii) *Osteitis pubis.*
b. *Tuberculous sacro-iliitis and osteitis pubis.*

The right sacro-iliac joint surfaces are indistinct, with subchondral erosion and sclerosis (Fig. 1.16a). There is loss of bone substance, irregularity and sclerosis on both sides of the symphysis pubis, which has dislocated.
    Sacro-iliitis is seen in a number of other conditions:

1. Ankylosing spondylitis: symmetrical. 90% of cases occur in men.
2. Reiter's disease: more often asymmetrical than in ankylosing spondylitis.
3. Psoriasis: in 30% of cases. Usually symmetrical, and associated with arthritis mutilans.
4. Inflammatory bowel disease.
5. Brucellosis: unilateral.

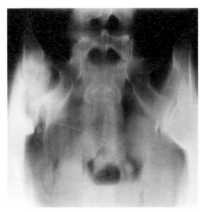

Fig. 1.16a
Tomogram of the sacro-iliac
joint in Q1.16

1.17

1. Fractured right clavicle.
2. Hydatid disease of the spleen.

There is a circular calcified mass below the left diaphragm. Infection with *Taenia echinococcus* is typically acquired in childhood in underdeveloped countries, usually through contact with the faeces of infected dogs, cattle or sheep. The usually solitary cyst occurs most frequently in the right lobe of the liver (Fig. 1.6a), but may also be found in the lung.

Other causes of splenic calcification are:

1. Tuberculosis or histoplasmosis: multiple, small, rounded, healed foci.
2. Calcified splenic infarcts, or splenic artery aneurysms.
3. Simple splenic cyst.
4. Post-traumatic splenic haemorrhage.
5. Chronic brucellosis (rare): multiple, large (1–3 cm) cysts, with calcified centres and rims with an intervening radiolucent area.

1.18

1. Renal tubular acidosis.
2. Hypercalcaemia (e.g. primary hyperparathyroidism, sarcoidosis).
3. Medullary sponge kidney.

Orderly calcification within solid renal tissue may be divided into two groups, according to which compartment it is in:

1. Medullary (as in this case): the causes are listed above. In renal papillary necrosis, a dense rim of calcification around the tip of each pyramid may occur.
2. Cortical: acute cortical necrosis (thin rim of calcification outlining the outer margin of one or both kidneys), chronic glomerulonephritis (rare), and chronic transplant rejection.

More patchy calcification in the kidney implies focal tissue damage, such as in tuberculosis (40% of cases), renal cell carcinoma (10% of cases), hydatid disease and amyloidosis.

1.19

Spinal angioma.

Tortuous ('serpiginous') filling defects are seen in the contrast medium, due to dilated vessels on the surface of the cord. They may cause spinal subarachnoid haemorrhage or spinal cord compression. A cutaneous angioma is present in 15% of cases, and may help localize the spinal lesion.

1.20

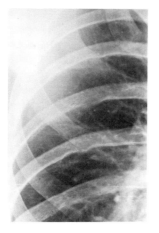

Fig. 1.20a
Coarctation: rib notching

a. *(i)* *Bilateral rib notching, affecting the lower borders of the fourth to eighth ribs (Dock's sign).*
   (ii) *Cardiomegaly with prominence of the left heart border, suggesting left ventricular hypertrophy.*
b. *Classical coarctation of the aorta, that is, the stenosis is opposite the origin of the ductus arteriosus.*

The rib notching (Fig. 1.20a) is caused by dilated tortuous intercostal arteries acting as collaterals, carrying blood retrogradely from each subclavian artery, which arise proximal to the coarctation, to the thoracic aorta distal to the stenosis. Rib notching will occur on the right side only, if the coarctation involves, or is proximal to, the origin of the left subclavian artery. Rib notching is rarely present until adolescence, and slowly disappears following surgical treatment of the coarctation. Other X-ray changes which may be seen in this condition include evidence of left ventricular hypertrophy, a dilated left subclavian artery above an apparently small aortic knuckle, or poststenotic dilatation of the descending aorta.

Rib notching, although characteristic of this condition, is not pathognomonic and has a number of other, rare causes:

1. Enlarged intercostal arteries: severe atheroma or thrombosis of the abdominal aorta (notching of the lower three ribs); subclavian artery obstruction (unilateral notching of the upper 3–4 ribs); Blalock–Taussig operation of subclavian-pulmonary artery anastomosis for Fallot's tetralogy (notching of the right upper 3–4 ribs).
2. Enlarged intercostal veins: superior or inferior vena cava obstruction.
3. Enlarged intercostal nerves: neurofibromatosis.

Section 2

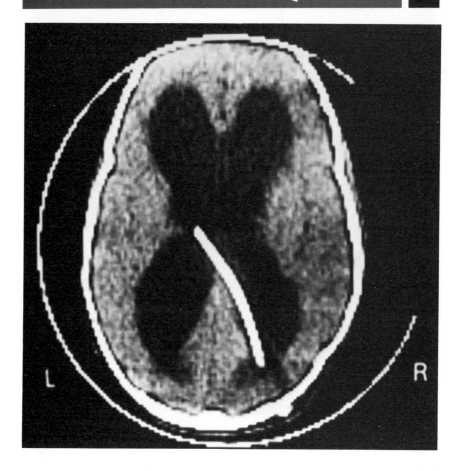

2.1

What are the causes of the two abnormalities visible on this CT scan?

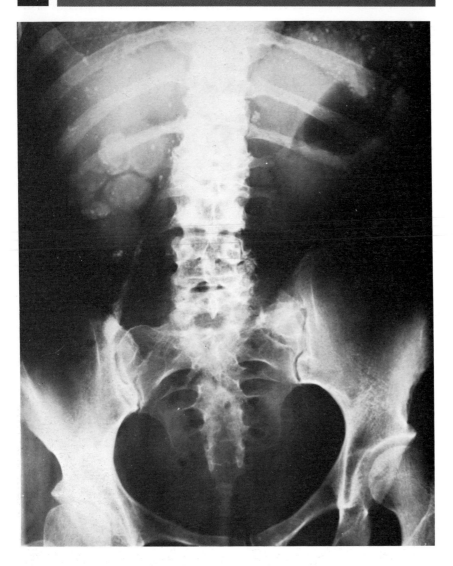

2.2

a. *Describe three abnormalities visible on this X-ray.*

b. *What is the cause of all of these changes?*

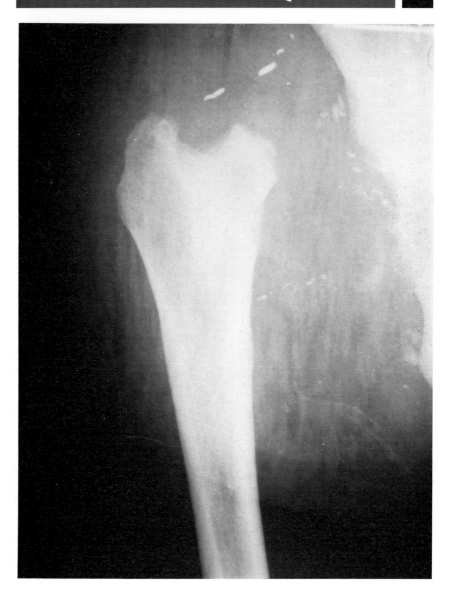

2.3

a. Describe two abnormalities seen on this X-ray of a 65-year-old man's hip joint.

b. What is the most likely cause of these changes?

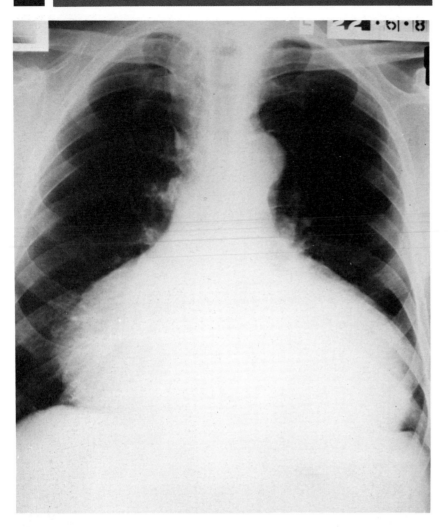

2.4

a. What is the diagnosis?

b. How may this be confirmed non-invasively?

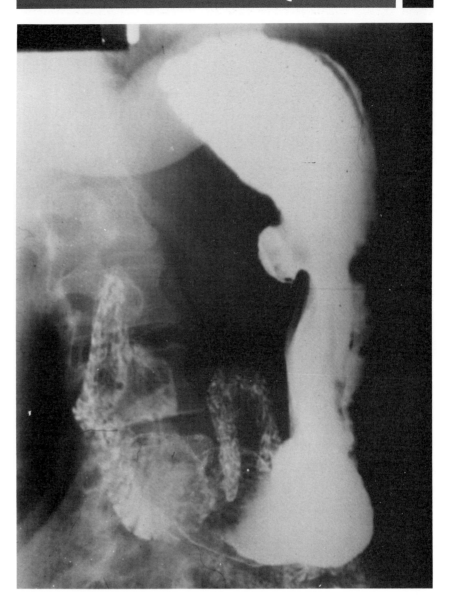

2.5
What is the diagnosis?

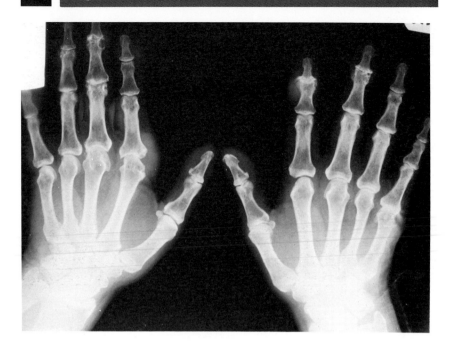

2.6

This 60-year-old man gives a history of joint pain:

a. Describe two abnormalities visible on this X-ray.
b. What is the diagnosis?

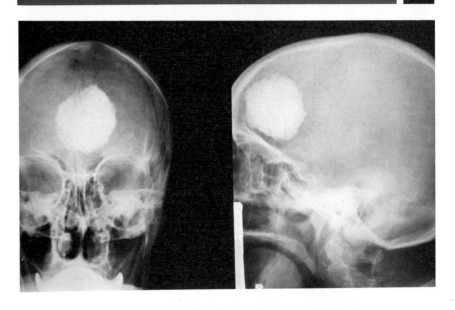

2.7
What is the diagnosis?

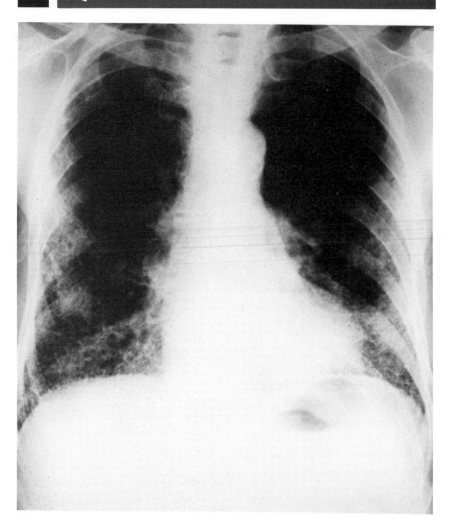

2.8

This elderly man presents with a 3-month history of increasing dyspnoea on exertion.

What is the cause of his symptoms?

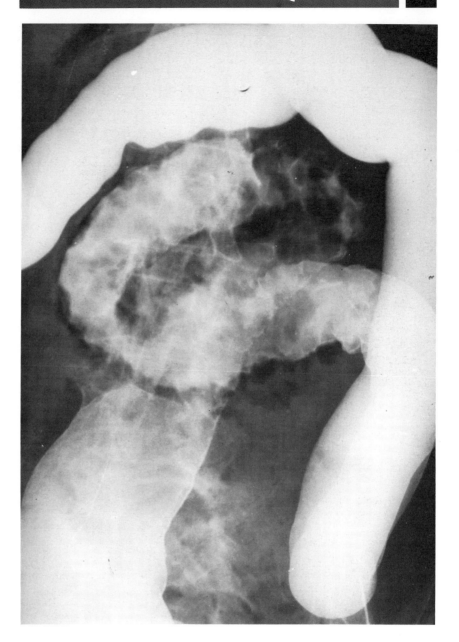

2.9

This is part of the barium enema of a man with chronic bronchitis, who gave a history of mild diarrhoea and episodic colicky abdominal pain.

What is the diagnosis?

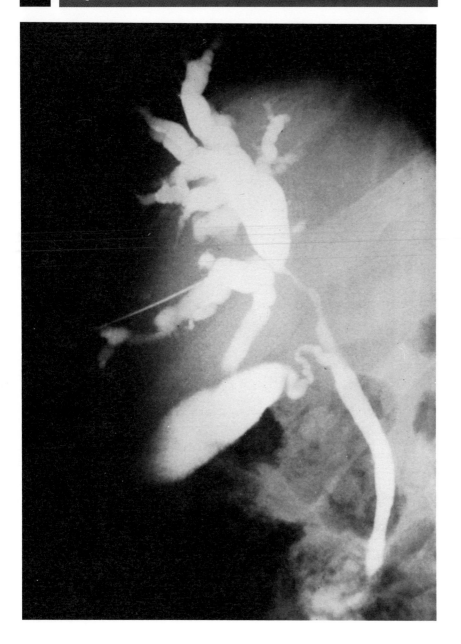

2.10

a. *What investigation is shown?*
b. *What two abnormalities are visible?*

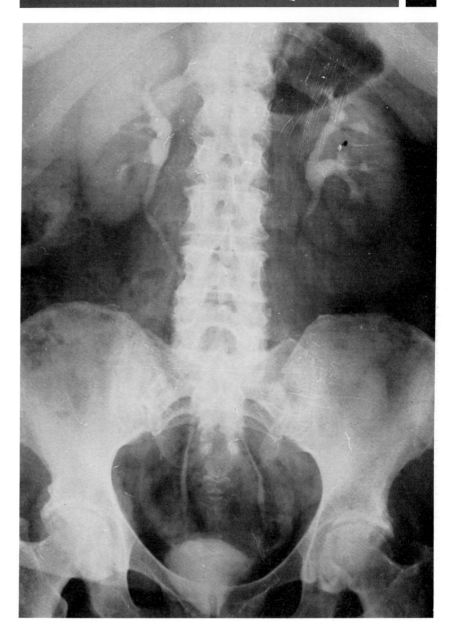

2.11

a. *Describe the abnormality seen on this X-ray.*
b. *What is the cause of this abnormality?*

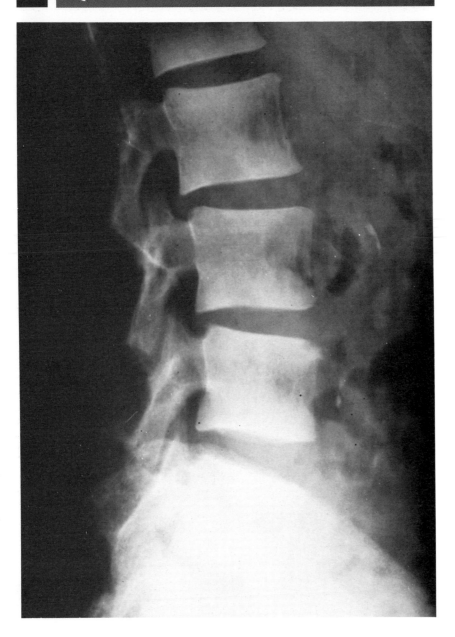

2.12

a. *What is the condition that has resulted in the changes visible on this X-ray of a 30-year-old man?*

b. *Name two other skeletal changes that may be seen in this condition.*

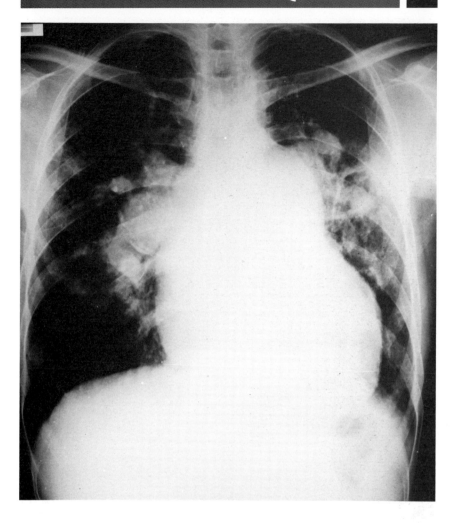

2.13

This 50-year-old man has heart failure.

a. What three abnormalities are visible on this film?
b. What is the cause of these changes?

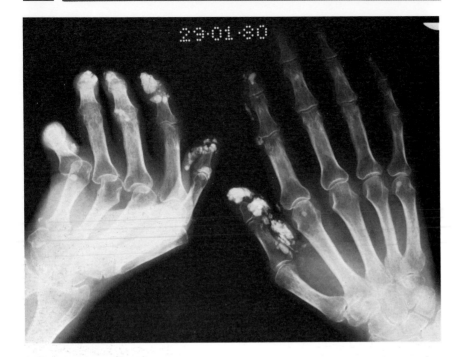

2.14

These hand X-rays are of a 60-year-old woman with pulmonary fibrosis.

a. What is the diagnosis?
b. What other radiological feature may be found in this disorder?

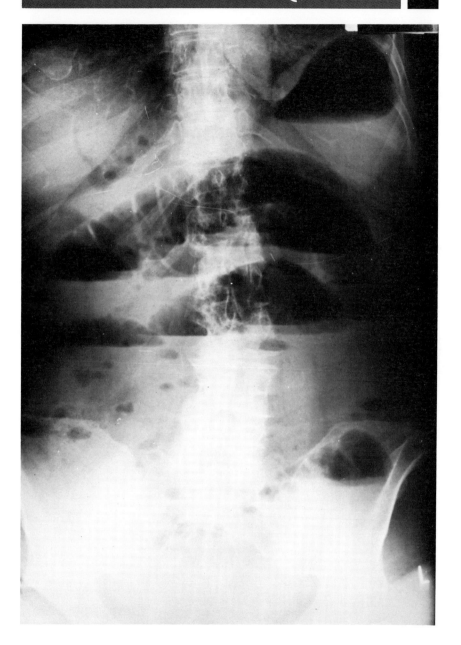

2.15

a. *What two sets of abnormalities are visible on this abdominal X-ray?*
b. *What is the diagnosis?*

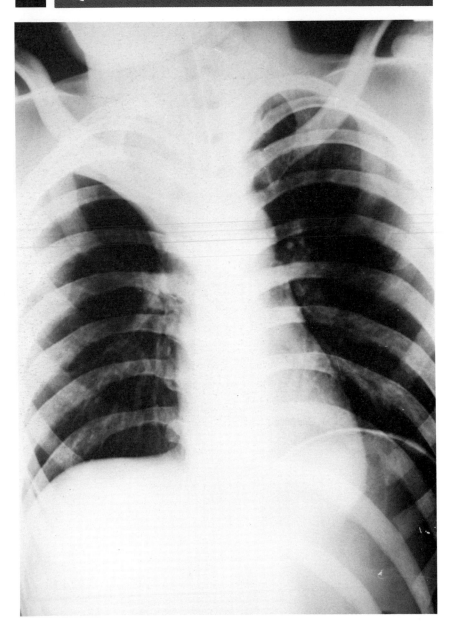

2.16

This man has acute asthma, and is on a ventilator.

What is the cause of his abnormal chest X-ray?

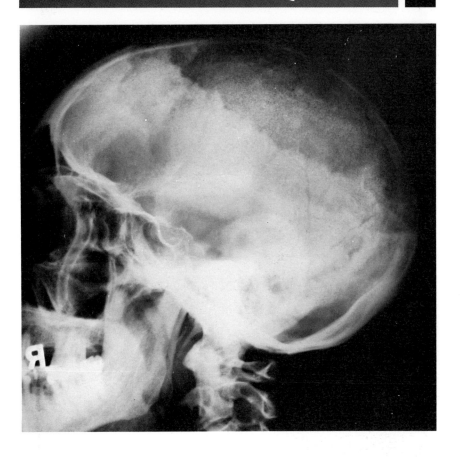

2.17

This is the skull X-ray of a 70-year-old man.

What is the diagnosis?

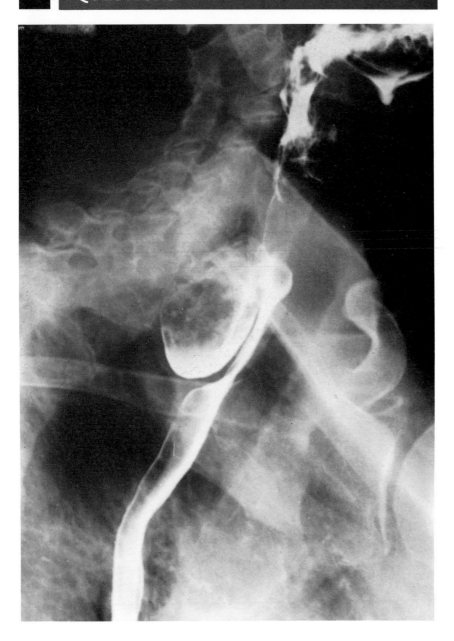

2.18

What is the cause of the abnormality visible on this X-ray?

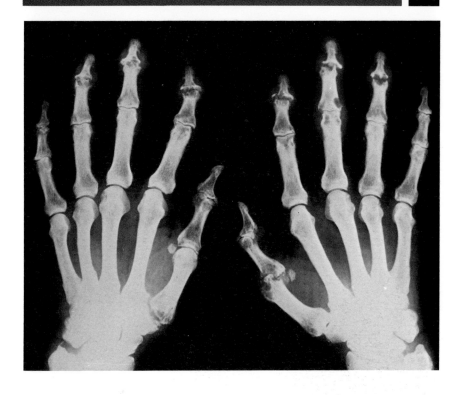

2.19

What is the most probable diagnosis?

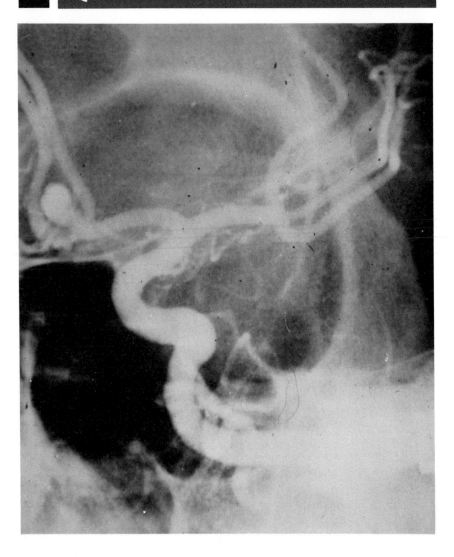

2.20

a. *What is the site of the abnormality shown on this carotid angiogram?*

b. *With what two congenital disorders may this abnormality be associated?*

2.1

1. *Hydrocephalus.*
2. *Ventricular shunt in situ.*

The cerebral ventricles are markedly dilated. In addition, there is a paraventricular rim of low attenuation suggesting active and acute hydrocephalus.

2.2

a. (i) *Calcification in the right upper quadrant outlining the collecting system in a pyonephrosis with autonephrectomy.*
   (ii) *Calcification in the line of the psoas sheath within a psoas abscess.*
   (iii) *Numerous small calcified foci throughout the liver and spleen, reflecting previous miliary disease.*
b. *Tuberculosis.*

There is evidence of previous extensive intra-abdominal tuberculosis, with involvement of the right kidney, liver and spleen.

Unlike pulmonary tuberculosis, the incidence of genitourinary tuber-culosis has remained steady for the past 30 years. It accounts for 2–3% of cases of tuberculosis in the United Kingdom. Early lesions might present as a slight irregularity of a minor calyx. Irregular cavities and calyceal cicatrization represent more advanced disease. Involvement of the ureter leads to fibrosis with stricture formation, and subsequent obstruction with atrophy of the kidney. Vesical involvement leads to a reduction in bladder capacity.

Prostatic, epididymal, and seminal vesicle calcification may also be seen.

With antituberculous chemotherapy, healing may result in stenosis (e.g. pyocalyx, pelvi-ureteric junction stricture, or ureteric obstruction). Follow-up intravenous urograms are therefore mandatory to detect these compli-cations early, and then treat appropriately (e.g. ureteric reimplantation).

2.3

a. (i) *The head of the femur has been totally destroyed. The margin of the defect is clearly defined, without osteoporosis. Within the joint space are numerous pieces of calcified debris (fragments of bone).*

   (ii) *Streaks of higher radiodensity above and below the joint, from previous intramuscular bismuth injections (A1.2).*

b. *Neuropathic or Charcot joint. Involvement of the hip joint suggests tabes dorsalis.*

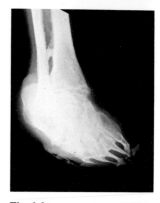

Fig. 2.3a
Leprosy: neuropathic foot.
Destroyed ('whittled') phalanges.
No calcified nerves are visible

The appearance of this atrophic type of neuropathic joint simulates surgical excision of the head and neck of the femur. In the hypertrophic form, more florid bony overgrowth of the joint margins, especially in the spine, may lead to confusion with the seronegative spondylarthropathies or osteoarthrosis. A neuropathic shoulder, elbow or wrist joint suggests syringomyelia. Neuropathic feet suggest diabetes or leprosy (Fig. 2.3a). Neuropathic hands also suggest leprosy (calcification of peripheral nerves may also be seen).

2.4

a. *Pericardial effusion.*
b. *Echocardiography will demonstrate an echo-free zone behind the left ventricle, and also often in front of the right ventricle.*

There is a massive, symmetrical enlargement of the heart ('globular' or 'flask-shaped') with a disproportionate enlargement inferiorly in the transverse diameter as compared to the increase in the vertical diameter. For the degree of apparent cardiomegaly the lung fields are remarkably clear. There is also an azygous lobe present.

Acute myocarditis, dilated (congestive) cardiomyopathy and marked biventricular enlargement (e.g. ventricular shunts, chronic rheumatic heart disease) can produce similar radiological features. They may also be complicated by pericardial effusion, and it may then be necessary to carry out contrast studies to differentiate the various conditions.

2.5
Gastric ulcer.

There is a large benign gastric ulcer on the lesser curve. It has many features to distinguish it from a malignant ulcer. There is a smooth base; the crater projects outside the normal lumen; there is a translucent halo or collar (oedema) around the orifice (Hampton's line); the edges of the crater are slightly undermined; and it is on the lesser rather than the greater curve. One feature, not visible in this view, is that in benign ulcers the gastric folds extend into the ulcer crater.

Despite these features, every gastric ulcer must be regarded with suspicion. Unsuspected malignancy is found in 5% of gastrectomy specimens. An early diagnosis of malignant change in an ulcer has a good prognosis with surgical treatment (60% 5-year survival). Where facilities exist, therefore, patients should be gastroscoped and malignancy excluded (in 99.5% of cases) by a combination of macroscopic appearances, histology (at least six biopsy specimens around the ulcer) and cytological brush samples.

2.6

a.   (i)   *Eccentric soft tissue swellings around the distal interphalangeal (DIP) and metacarpophalangeal (MCP) joints of the left index finger, and the DIP joint of the right index finger.*

   (ii) *'Punched-out' lesion near the distal end of the middle phalanx of the left middle finger. This has clearly defined endosteal margins.*

b.   *Gouty arthropathy.*

Radiologically, the main distinction is from rheumatoid disease:

1. In gout, the soft tissue swellings (tophi) are eccentric, and may calcify. Symmetrical joint swelling is seen in rheumatoid disease, unless a nodule overlies the joint, and calcification is not seen.
2. The erosive changes in gout are due to deposition of urate crystals. They are characteristically large, with clearly defined edges. Furthermore, they are usually juxta-articular in distribution and, as they enlarge, involve more of the cortex of the shaft than the articular surface. In some cases, intra-osseous calcification is seen. In contrast, rheumatoid erosions are due to inflammatory overgrowth of the synovium (pannus), and affect the articular surfaces of the joint. They are often small, with indistinct margins, and do not calcify.
3. Gouty joints have less marked periarticular osteoporosis.
4. Gout tends to attack the distal and proximal interphalangeal (PIP) joints, whereas rheumatoid disease affects the MCP and PIP joints.

Clinically, these conditions are easily differentiated. The diagnosis of gout is never established initially by radiology, as erosive changes do not appear until there is clinical evidence of tophi.

   Radiological differentiation from Ollier's disease (multiple enchondromata — Fig. 2.6a) may also be difficult.

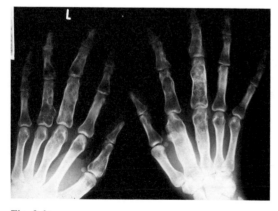

Fig. 2.6a
Ollier's disease: the
endochromata tend to spare the
bone ends

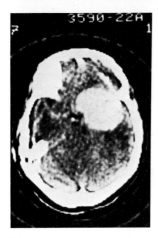

Fig. 2.7a
Enhanced CT scan: meningioma
in the region of the left
sphenoidal ridge

2.7

Calcified falx meningioma.

Calcified meningiomas frequently show this characteristic, well-defined 'ball of calcium'. The parasagittal site (originating from the superior sagittal sinus) should also suggest this diagnosis. Meningiomas account for 15% of primary brain tumours. 95% are benign, and 20% calcify. They are thought to arise from the arachnoid cells of the arachnoid villi, and so are commonly found along the course of the intracranial venous sinuses, namely the superior sagittal sinus (50%), sphenoidal ridge (Fig. 2.7a), the convexity of the hemispheres and the suprasellar region. About half the patients with intracranial meningiomas have an abnormal plain skull X-ray.

There are a number of other causes of pathological intracranial calcification:

1. Other tumours: appears as a dense nodule, a few ill-defined specks, or irregular linear or serpiginous streaks.
   a. Gliomas: 5–10% calcify, especially oligodendrogliomas.
   b. Craniopharyngioma: 75% calcify; characteristic position in the midline, just above the sella.
   c. Ependymoma, pinealoma, choroid plexus papilloma, pituitary adenoma (very rare).
2. Vascular lesions:
   a. Aneurysm: marginal calcification.
   b. Angioma: flecks of calcification.
   c. Chronic subdural haematoma: calcification outlines the subdural membrane.
3. Infections and infestations:
   a. Tuberculosis: tuberculoma, or healed basal meningitis.
   b. Toxoplasmosis: multiple flecks in the cortex, and linear streaks in the basal ganglia.
   c. Cysticercosis.
   d. Pyogenic abscess.
4. Miscellaneous:
   a. Hypoparathyroidism: basal ganglia.
   b. Tuberose sclerosis: multiple, discrete rounded shadows.
   c. Sturge–Weber syndrome: parallel sinuous lines conforming to the distribution and shape of the cerebral sulci and gyri (associated with facial naevi).

2.8

Pulmonary fibrosis.

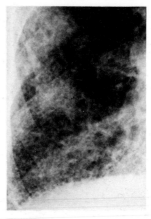

There are prominent interstitial markings at both bases. In places, the criss-crossing fine linear shadows resemble a honeycomb or fine cystic pattern (Fig. 2.8a). In other parts there are more nodular changes with areas of patchy consolidation. In more advanced cases, there may be radiological evidence of loss of lung volume (elevation of diaphragm, or fissure), bullae formation, and pulmonary arterial hypertension.

Though characteristic of fibrosis, these findings do not distinguish between the large number of cases of this disorder. A honeycomb pattern is especially seen in cryptogenic fibrosing alveolitis, scleroderma, asbestosis, rheumatoid lung and bronchiectasis.

Fig. 2.8a
Pulmonary fibrosis

Other radiological features might help differentiate the various causes of pulmonary fibrosis, for example:

1. Distribution: predominantly lower lobe fibrosis is seen in asbestosis and scleroderma, whereas in bird-fancier's lung and bronchopulmonary aspergillosis there is usually upper lobe involvement.
2. Asbestos-related pleural plaques: characteristic 'holly-leaf' pleural plaques or calcified plaques on the diaphragm (Fig. 2.8b) may be seen in asbestosis. Such plaques are more easily seen on computed tomography of the chest (Fig. 2.8c).
3. Pleural effusion: occurs especially in lymphangitis carcinomatosa, lymphomas, rheumatoid lung and systemic lupus erythematosus. Rare in cryptogenic fibrosing alveolitis, sarcoidosis and scleroderma.
4. Hilar lymphadenopathy: seen in sarcoidosis, silicosis and fungal infections.

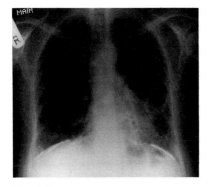

Fig. 2.8b
Asbestos-related pleural plaques:
calcified plaques on diaphragm
and, *en face*, in left mid-zone, in
a case of asbestosis

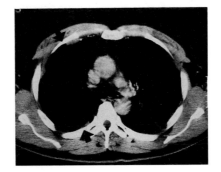

Fig. 2.8c
CT scan: pleural plaques (in
places calcified) lining the inside
of the hemithorax (arrowed)

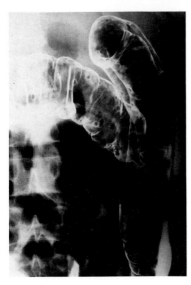
Fig. 2.9a
Familial polyposis coli

2.9

Pneumatosis cystoides intestinalis.

The wall of a short length of large bowel contains numerous air-filled cysts. This uncommon disorder affects two distinct age groups:

1. Infants under one year: associated with pyloric stenosis and intestinal obstruction. Gas is thought to pass from the lumen through breaches in the mucosa. The prognosis is related to the underlying gut disorder. It is also reported in older children with juvenile chronic arthritis, and after steroid therapy.
2. Adults: cysts develop (a) during colitis or bowel infarction; (b) following endoscopy; (c) in scleroderma, polymyositis, and chronic obstructive airways disease. In the latter, air is thought to leak into the retroperitoneal space from the lung and track down to the bowel wall. Cysts may be symptomless, or cause non-specific symptoms as in this case. They may be complicated by pneumoperitoneum. The prognosis is usually good, the cysts regressing spontaneously.

Differentiation from multiple intestinal polyps is usually easy. These may occur in a number of syndromes:

1. Familial polyposis coli (Fig. 2.9a): autosomal dominant. Between 2000 and 5000 adenomas develop in the large bowel, usually during the second or third decade of life. Carcinomas arise in all cases, about 10 years after the adenomas develop. Treatment is by total colectomy and ileo-rectal anastomosis.
2. Gardner's syndrome: multiple adenomas arise in the large bowel, and are premalignant. Associated with multiple skull osteomata, epidermoid cysts and soft tissue tumours of the skin.
3. Peutz–Jeghers syndrome: numerous hamartomas, which are not premalignant, in the small and large (50%) bowel. Associated with circumoral and mucosal pigmentation.

Linear streaks of gas in the intestinal wall are occasionally seen in ischaemic colitis. In necrotizing enterocolitis of infancy both linear and cystic collections of gas may be seen. Streaks of gas may also be seen in the wall of the bladder or gall bladder ('emphysematous cholecystitis') in associated with infections (especially in diabetes).

2.10

a. Percutaneous transhepatic cholangiogram.
b.   (i) Dilated intrahepatic ducts.
*   (ii) Stricture of the common hepatic duct.*

The abnormalities seen in this case were secondary to extrinsic compression of the common hepatic duct by enlarged lymph nodes (metastases) in the hilum of the liver.

Endoscopic retrograde choledochopancreatography (ERCP) also allows contrast imaging of the biliary tract (Fig. 2.10a).

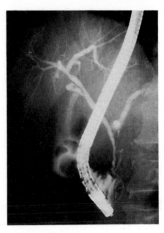

Fig. 2.10a
ERCP: stricture of proximal end of pancreatic duct (with dilatation distally), and gall stones in the gall bladder

2.11

a. Medial deviation of the lower part of each ureter.
b. Abdominoperineal resection.

In contrast, in retroperitoneal fibrosis, there is medial deviation of the upper part of the ureter (usually starting with a sharp 'medial hitch'), with variable dilatation of the calyces, pelvis and ureter. The fibrous tissue envelops the aorta and inferior vena cava, starting at the level of the renal pedicle and ending abruptly at the pelvic brim. It extends laterally beyond the outer margins of the psoas muscle. There are many causes of this disorder:

1. Benign (70%):
   a. Drugs: methysergide, ergot.
   b. Foreign material in the peritoneum: blood (leaking aortic aneurysm), kidney (renal rupture).
   c. Inflammation: Crohn's disease, actinomycoses, ischiorectal abscess.
   d. Idiopathic (commonest).
2. Malignant (30%): fibrosis is often confined to the pelvis:
   a. Pelvic neoplasms: rectum, female genital tract.
   b. Carcinoma (breast, bronchus, prostate, testicular) or lymphoma.

In muscular subjects and Africans, normal ureters may deviate medially at the level of the fourth or fifth lumbar vertebrae.

2.12

a. Renal (uraemic) osteodystrophy. There are bands of increased bone density within the vertebral bodies, which alternate with relatively less dense intervening bands ('rugger-jersey spine'). In addition, there is metastatic calcification of the wall of the abdominal aorta.

b. (i) Osteomalacia or rickets.
(ii) Hyperparathyroidism.
(iii) Osteoporosis.

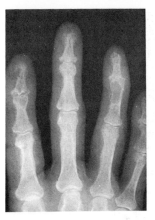

Fig. 2.12a
Hyperparathyroidism: subperiosteal erosions on the radial side of the phalanges, resorption of the distal phalangeal tufts, and a 'brown tumour' in the shaft of the middle phalanx of the index and ring fingers

The pathognomonic radiological sign of excess circulating parathormone is subperiosteal resorption. This is best seen on the radial surfaces of the proximal and middle phalanges of the hand (Fig. 2.12a). There may also be resorption of the tufts of the distal phalanges, the distal end of the clavicle and at sites of muscle insertions (e.g. ischial tuberosities). In addition, large cystic-like 'brown tumours' may be seen in the phalanges, metacarpals, and long bones. The skull often has a mottled, ground-glass appearance.

2.13

a. (i) Marked dilatation of the pulmonary trunk and central pulmonary arteries ('deer's antlers'), with 'pruning' of the peripheral pulmonary vasculature.
(ii) Calcification of the main branches of the pulmonary arteries.
(iii) Cardiomegaly, with evidence to suggest enlargement of both the right atrium (cardiac silhouette projects further to the right of the spine than normal) and ventricle (the apex is elevated above the diaphragm).
b. Pulmonary arterial hypertension.

Pulmonary arterial calcification reflects the chronicity of the hypertension in this case of a secundum atrial septal defect.
  Pulmonary arterial hypertension may be due to:

1. Hyperkinetic causes: increased pulmonary blood flow (intracardiac shunt; hyperdynamic circulation).
2. Pulmonary arterial vasoconstriction: hypoxia (chronic obstructive airways disease, high altitude), drugs (aminorex), or pulmonary venous hypertension (mitral stenosis, left ventricular failure).
3. Arterial obliteration: emboli (thrombus, tumour), parasites (*Schistosoma*), emphysema, or pulmonary fibrosis.
4. Idiopathic or primary pulmonary hypertension.

2.14

a. *Progressive or diffuse systemic sclerosis (scleroderma).*

b. *An aperistaltic, somewhat dilated oesophagus on barium swallow. The small and large intestine may be similarly affected. Rarer features include resorption of the distal end of the calvicle and pneumatosis cystoides intestinalis.*

There is extensive subcutaneous calcification, loss of soft tissue at the tips of the fingers (poikiloderma), and flexion deformities of the fingers of the left hand (due to the tight skin). Similar changes may be seen in the CREST syndrome, but the presence of pulmonary fibrosis suggests more systemic disease. There are numerous other causes of soft tissue calcification:

1. Vessels: atheroma (old age, diabetes, renal failure), varicose veins.
2. Nerves: leprosy, neurofibromatosis.
3. Metabolic: hypercalcaemia, renal failure, gout (tophi).
4. Haematomas.
5. Soft tissue necrosis: Ehlers–Danlos syndrome (subcutaneous oval lesions, which look like pheboliths), polymyositis (particularly in children; sheets of intramuscular calcification), intramuscular injections (quinine, gold).
6. Parasitic calcification: cysticercosis, Loa-loa (Fig. 2.14a).
7. Traumatic: fracture, burns.
8. Lymph nodes: tuberculosis.
9. Paraplegia: neuropathic joints (A2.3); myositis ossificans.
10. Calcified soft tissue tumours.
11. Radio-opaque material: failed arthrogram (spillage of dye into the soft tissues), intramuscular injections of bismuth (A2.3).

Surface absorption of the tip of the terminal phalanx may also be seen in a number of conditions:

1. Pyogenic infection (one digit only).
2. Neuropathic joint (Fig. 2.3a).
3. Traumatic amputation (one digit only).
4. Raynaud's phenomenon (Fig. 2.14b), frost bite, Buerger's disease.
5. Arthritis mutilans (rheumatoid disease, psoriatic arthropathy).
6. Hyperparathyroidism.
7. Bone sarcoid.
8. Polyvinyl chloride poisoning.
9. Progeria.

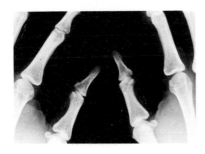

Fig. 2.14a
Loa-loa

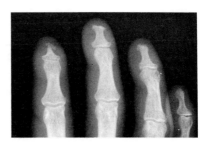

Fig. 2.14b
Raynaud's phenomenon:
resorption of the tips of the
terminal phalanges

2.15

a. (i) *Small bowel obstruction: there are numerous distended loops of small bowel (recognizable by their complete transverse bands: valvulae conniventes), containing fluid levels, with small gas bubbles in the more distal bowel ('string of beads').*
    (ii) *Air in the biliary tree.*
b. *Gall-stone ileus.*

This is usually caused by a gall stone eroding through the wall of the inflamed gall bladder, into the adjacent duodenum. The stone, although large enough to cause an incomplete obstruction in the distal ileum, may not be sufficiently calcified to be seen.

Air in the biliary tree may also be seen following damage to the sphincter of Oddi (operation, passage of a stone, or tumour), and in gas-forming infections in the biliary tract. This has to be differentiated from air in the portal veins (Fig. 2.15a), which is visible as smooth branches of translucency radiating to the liver edge. This is seen in necrotizing enterocolitis, mesenteric infarction, ingestion of corrosives and in gas embolus after bacterial endocarditis.

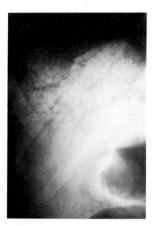

Fig. 2.15a
Air in the portal veins

2.16

Collapse of the right upper lobe, most probably secondary to mucous plug obstruction.

The characteristic radiological features of complete collapse of this lobe are shown. The horizontal (lesser) fissure is drawn upwards, and curved towards the apex and mediastinum. Above it is the radio-opaque collapsed lobe. There is compensatory spread of the lower and middle lobe vessels, and the lower pole of the elevated right hilum has swung outwards.

Each lobe collapses in a characteristic fashion (Figs 2.16a and 2.16b) resulting in one or more of the following: a radio-opacity, displacement of a fissure, compensatory overinflation, displacement of the hilum or mediastinum or diaphragm and the absence of an air bronchogram (often present in lobar pneumonia). Radiological clues as to the cause of the collapse may also be present; such as, bronchogenic tumour (adenoma, carcinoma), enlarged lymph nodes, tuberculosis (bronchostenosis), or an inhaled foreign body.

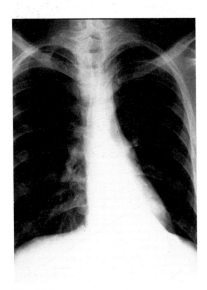

Fig. 2.16a
Left lower lobe collapse

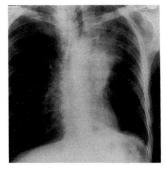

Fig. 2.16b
Left upper lobe collapse

2.17

Osteoporosis circumscripta.

In some cases of Paget's disease, the vault, instead of being thickened, shows a single area of relative translucency with thinning of the outer table. Its margin is sharply demarcated. In most cases there are typical radiological appearances of Paget's disease elsewhere. Other cases show more prominent thickening of the calvarium, with patchy sclerosis (Fig. 2.17a — 'cotton-wool' effect), and basilar invagination (platybasia). Neurological complications of this disease are cranial nerve palsies (especially the vestibulo-cochlear, olfactory and optic nerves), and spinal cord compression.

Generalized thickening of the skull vault may also be seen in acromegaly, osteopetrosis (Fig. 2.17b), thalassaemia major (Fig. 1.11a), dystrophia myotonica (small pituitary), and prolonged phenytoin therapy (widened diploë).

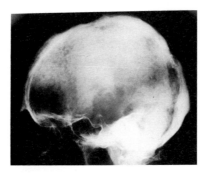

Fig. 2.17a
Paget's disease: 'woolly' skull

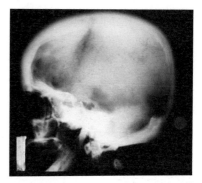

Fig. 2.17b
Osteopetrosis

2.18

Pharyngeal pouch (Zenker's diverticulum).

This is a pulsion diverticulum, the pharyngeal mucosa protruding through the dehiscence between the oblique and transverse fibres of the inferior constrictor muscle of the pharynx. The pouch projects posteriorly and usually to the left.

Clinically they manifest themselves with discomfort on swallowing or regurgitation of undigested food. Some present as a mass in the left side of the neck.

Diverticula may also occur in the mid-portion of the oesophagus ('traction diverticulum', associated with tuberculous mediastinal lymph nodes) and, less commonly, at the lower end of the oesophagus (epiphrenic), where they may be confused with a hiatus hernia.

2.19

Psoriatic arthropathy.

About 7% of patients with psoriasis have an arthropathy. This may take one of four forms:

1. Distal arthritis: an inflammatory arthropathy affecting the DIP joints of the fingers (of which 60–80% show nail involvement), and the interphalangeal joints of the toes (especially the big toe). Subchondral erosive lesions may be seen, often with considerable loss of bone ends (heads of middle phalanges, distal phalanges — Fig. 2.19a). Compared with rheumatoid disease, the arthropathy is more asymmetrical, there is less periarticular osteoporosis, and more periosteal new bone formation. This can result in marginal bony overgrowth at sites of tendon insertion (which may simulate Heberden's nodes). Bony ankylosis may develop early.
2. A symmetrical polyarthritis indistinguishable from rheumatoid disease, but persistently seronegative.
3. Arthritis mutilans: extensive resorption of the distal ends of phalanges gives them a whittled appearance ('licked candy-stick'), and results in telescoping of the now surplus soft tissue (*main-en-lorgnette* — opera-glass hand).
4. Sacro-iliitis with paraspinal ossification (30% of cases): this may occur alone, or with any of the other forms of psoriatic arthropathy (commoner with arthritis mutilans). The appearance in the sacro-iliac joints in non-specific, though more often asymmetrical. The paravertebral ossification, however, differs from ankylosing spondylitis in that it is characteristically separated from the vertebral body.

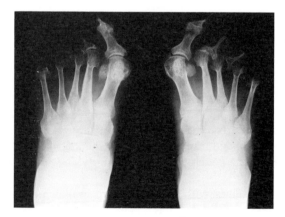

Fig. 2.19a
Psoriatic arthropathy: resorption of the heads of the proximal tarsal bones ('pencil deformity'), and almost complete resorption of the distal tarsal bones. Subluxation of the metatarsophalangeal joints

2.20

a. *Aneurysm at the junction of the anterior communicating and anterior cerebral arteries.*

b. (i) *Coarctation of the aorta.*
   (ii) *Polycystic disease of the kidneys, liver, or both (Figs 1.6b and 2.20a).*

This is the commonest site of intracranial aneurysm formation, accounting for 28% of cases. Other common sites are the origin of the posterior communicating artery (25%), the bifurcation of the main middle cerebral artery (20%), and the terminal segment of the internal carotid artery (6%). Multiple aneurysms are found in between 5 and 15% of cases.

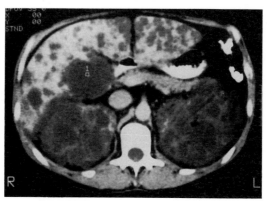

Fig. 2.20a
Abdominal CT: polycystic kidneys and multiple cysts in the liver, of which the largest is indicated by the cursor

Section 3

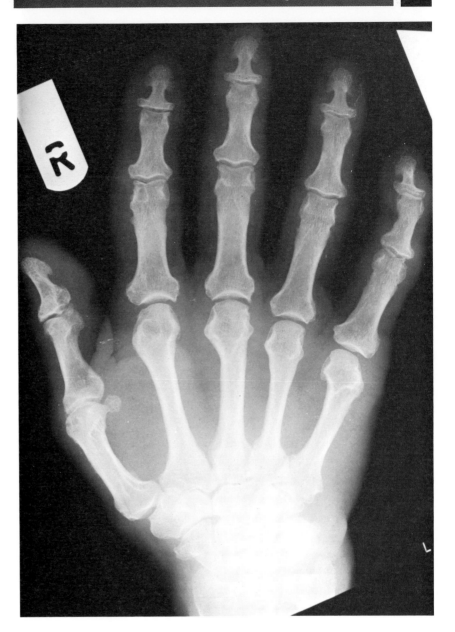

3.1

This man has visual impairment.

a. *What is the diagnosis?*
b. *Describe three other radiological features that may be present in this condition.*

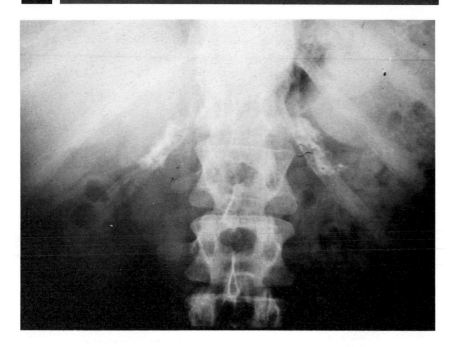

3.2

a. What abnormality is visible on this X-ray?
b. Suggest four possible causes of this finding.

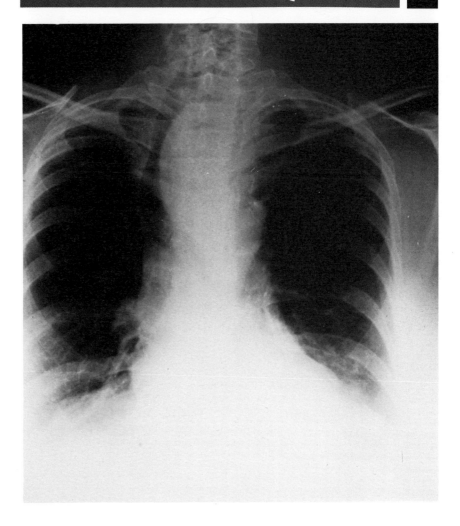

3.3

What is the cause of this 50-year-old lady's abnormal X-ray?

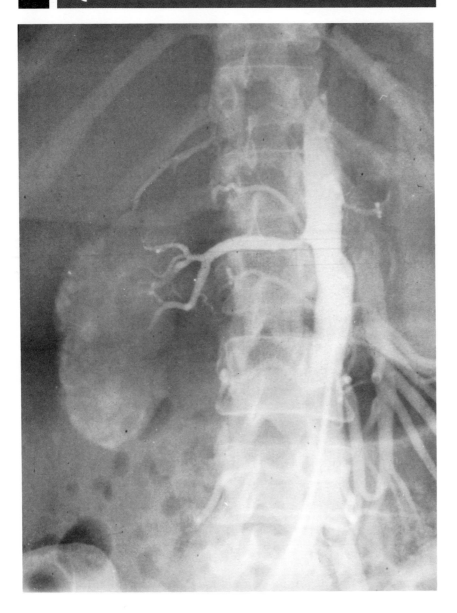

3.4

This renal arteriogram is of a 50-year-old man with hypertension.

a. What is the diagnosis?
b. Describe three abnormalities that would be seen in this kidney on the intravenous urogram (assuming the other side is normal).

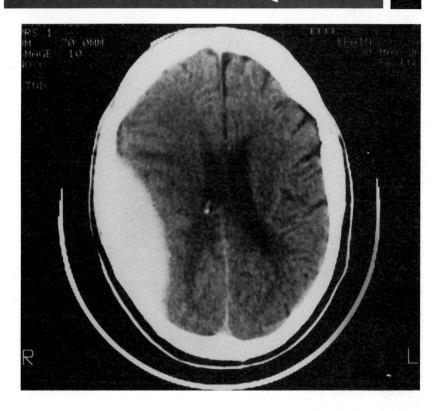

3.5

This man's conscious level deteriorated shortly after a head injury.

What is the diagnosis?

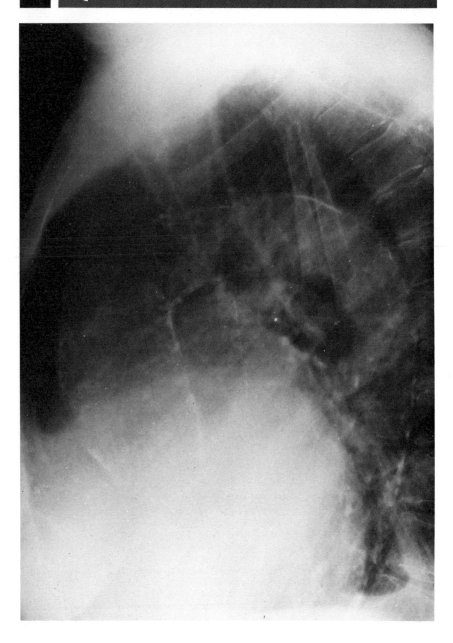

3.6

a. *What abnormality is visible on this X-ray?*

b. *What three pathological processes might cause this change?*

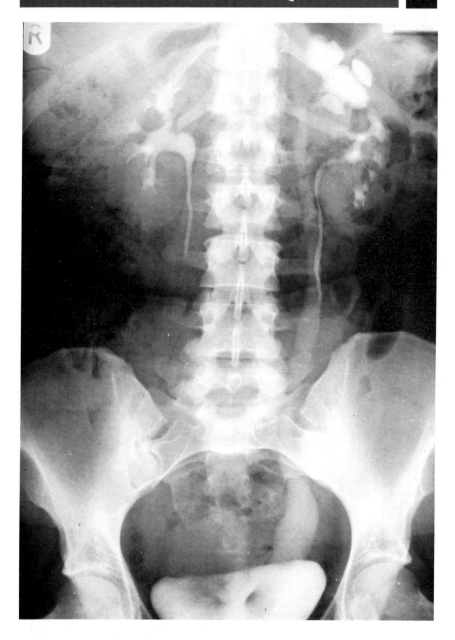

3.7

Describe four abnormalities seen on this intravenous urogram.

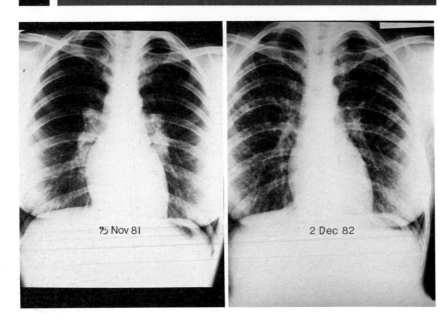

3.8

What is the diagnosis in this 40-year-old woman?

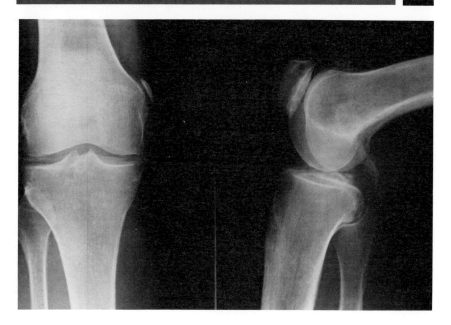

3.9

a. What is the diagnosis?
b. Name six conditions in which this abnormality may be found.

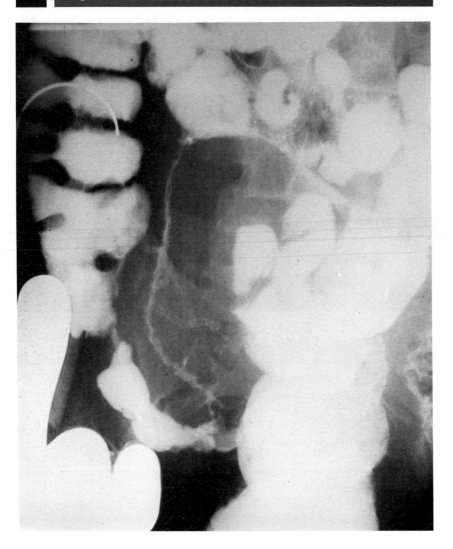

3.10

What is the diagnosis?

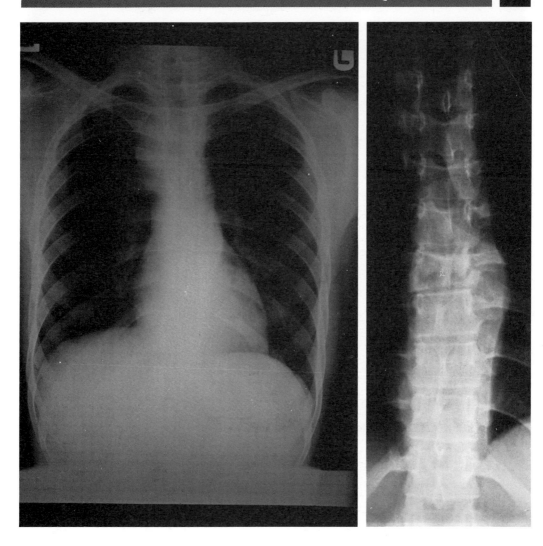

3.11

This young Indian man presented with a history of lethargy and back pain.

a. *What abnormality is visible on his chest X-ray?*
b. *What abnormality is visible on his thoracic spine X-ray?*
c. *What is the most likely diagnosis?*

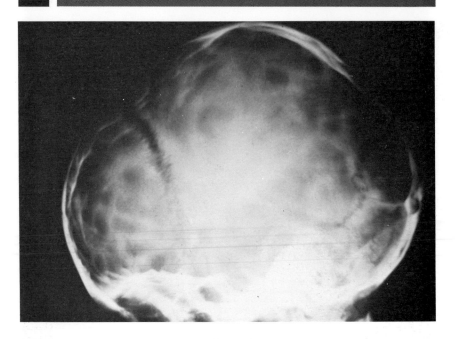

3.12

This 12-year-old girl has epilepsy.

a. Describe two abnormalities visible on her skull X-ray.
b. What is the most likely cause of these changes?

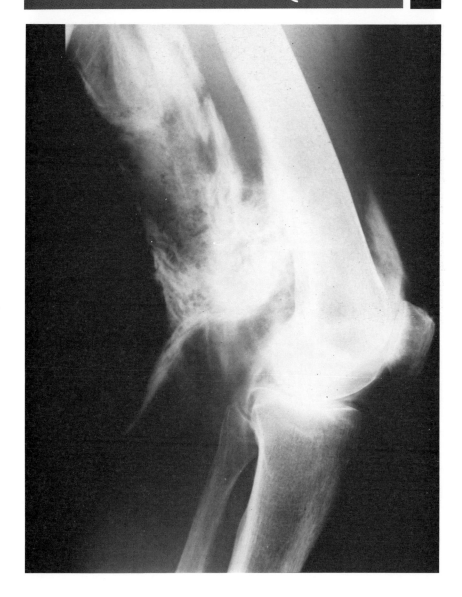

3.13
What is the diagnosis?

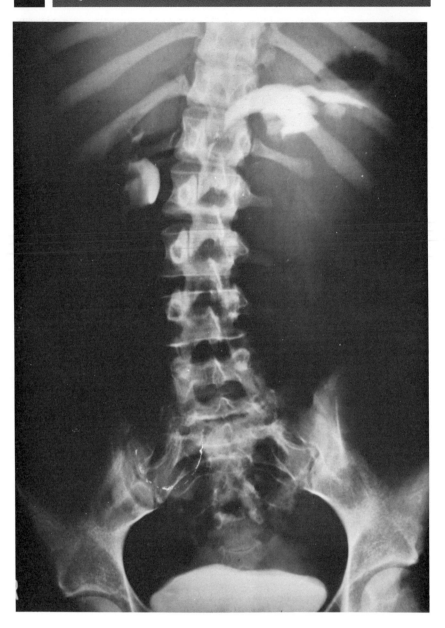

3.14

This 12-year-old girl presented with malignant hypertension and an abdominal mass.

a. What two abnormalities are visible on her intravenous urogram?
b. Give two possible diagnoses.

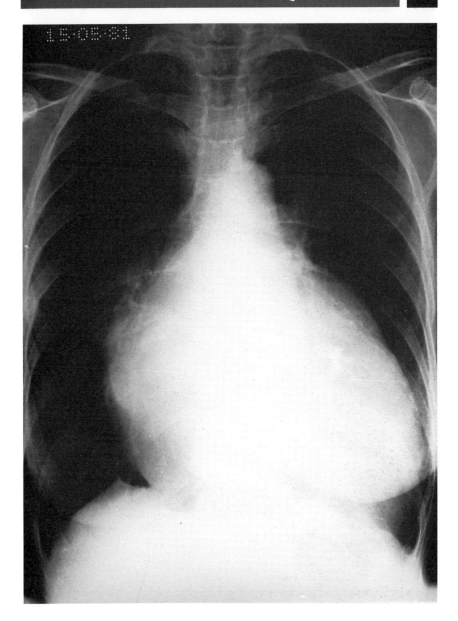

3.15
What two abnormalities are visible on this X-ray?

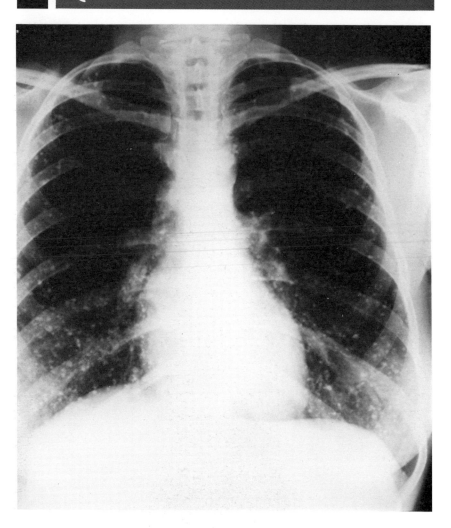

3.16

This is the chest X-ray of a 25-year-old man, taken during a routine medical examination.

What is the diagnosis?

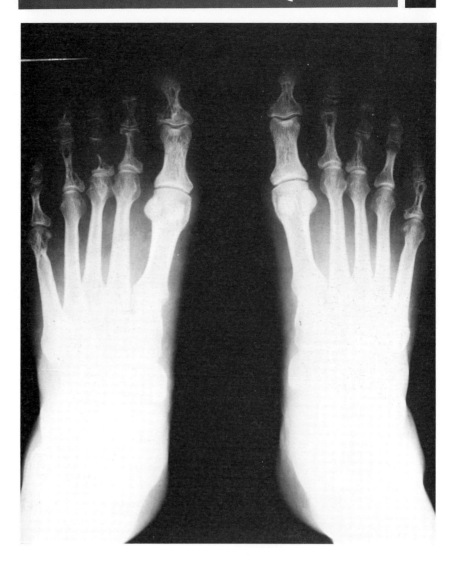

3.17

This negro man presented with a history of skin rash and pain in both feet.

a. Describe three abnormalities visible on his X-ray.
b. What is the diagnosis?

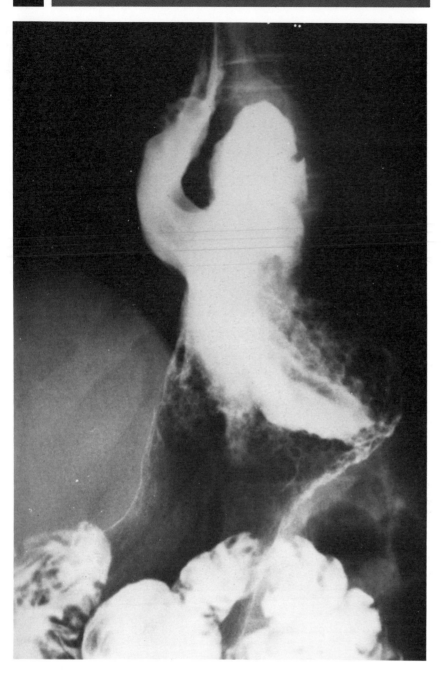

3.18

What is the diagnosis?

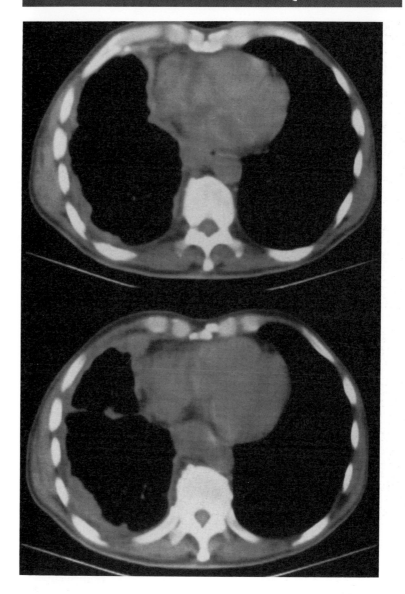

3.19

This 65-year-old retired dock labourer presents with a 3-month history of dull right-sided chest pain, increasing breathlessness and weight loss.

What is the most likely diagnosis?

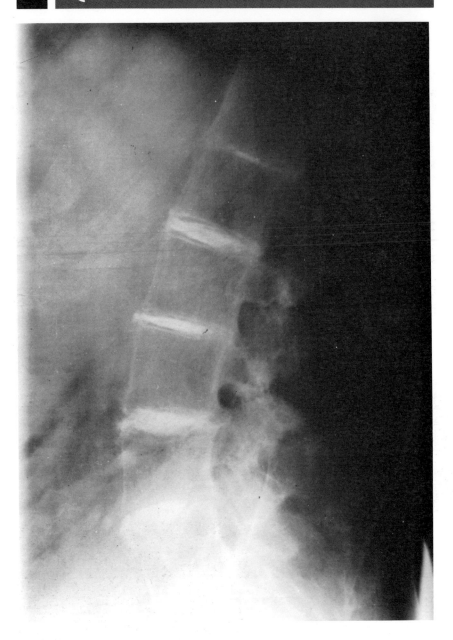

3.20

This 50-year-old man complains of low back pain.

a. What is the diagnosis?
b. Name two other symptoms that he might have noticed.

3.1

a. *Acromegaly. The hands are large ('spade-like') due to enlargement of all tissues (bone, cartilage, soft tissue). There is broadening of the distal phalangeal tufts, the joint margins and other bony ridges (sites of tendon or muscle attachment). The joint spaces of the MCP joints are widened due to excessive growth of cartilage.*

b.
   (i) *Similar changes may be seen in the feet (Fig. 3.1a). Bone overgrowth has caused 'beak-like' deformities of the heads of the first metatarsals.*

  (ii) *The skull is abnormal in 80% of cases (Fig. 3.1b). Typically, the vault is thickened, the frontal air sinuses enlarged, and there is uniform expansion of the sella. The size and angle of the mandible may be increased (prognathism), with reversed bite and separation of the teeth.*

 (iii) *A diagnostic feature is the thickness of the heel pad (Fig. 3.1c), usually less than 21.5 mm in female and 23 mm in male patients.*

 (iv) *Enlargement of the viscera (heart, kidneys or liver) may be evident.*

  (v) *Other radiological features include chondrocalcinosis, calcification within the pinna, an increase in the anteroposterior diameter of the vertebral bodies, kyphosis, osteoporosis, and changes of secondary osteoarthrosis.*

CT of the pituitary fossa (Fig. 3.1d) usually clearly demonstrates the presence or absence of a tumour.

If growth hormone hypersecretion occurs before epiphyseal fusion, gigantism results and may coexist with acromegaly. The severity of the radiological changes does not correlate well with growth hormone levels, but does with levels of plasma somatomedin.

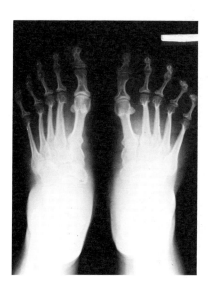

Fig. 3.1a
Acromegaly

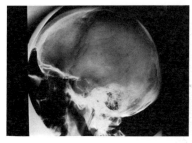

Fig. 3.1b
Acromegaly

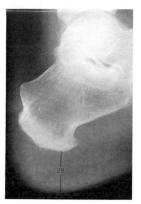

Fig. 3.1c
Acromegaly: heel pad
thickness — 28 mm

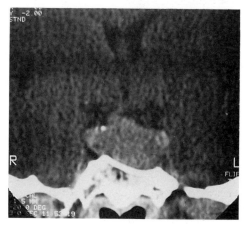

Fig. 3.1d
CT: coronal section of pituitary fossa showing
large hyperdense mass extending out of the fossa

3.2

a. Bilateral adrenal calcification.

b.   *(i)* *Consequence of adrenal haemorrhage during infancy: usually have normal adrenal function.*

    (ii) *Auto-immune Addison's disease.*

    (iii) *Tuberculosis.*

    (iv) *Neoplasms: phaeochromocytomas, neuroblastoma, adenoma, carcinoma.*

    (v) *Xanthomatosis, Niemann–Pick disease.*

In the upper abdomen, pancreatic calcification may also be seen. Diffuse calcification (Figs 3.2a and 3.2b) is a late and infrequent feature of chronic pancreatitis, and is due to the precipitation of calcium carbonate around protein plugs in the duct system. This may also be seen in cystic fibrosis, kwashiorkor, and hyperparathyroidism. More focal deposits of calcium may occur in pancreatic carcinomas and cysts.

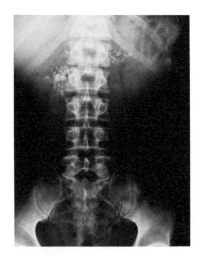

Fig. 3.2a
Calcification of the head, body and tail of the pancreas

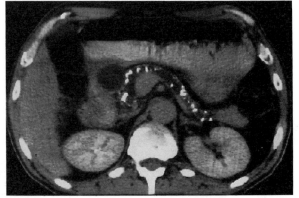

Fig. 3.2b
Enhanced CT scan: irregular dilatation of the pancreatic duct with multiple areas of calcification, and a cystic area in the head of the pancreas

3.3

Retrosternal goitre.

The characteristic X-ray features of this mediastinal tumour are shown (Figs 3.3a and 3.3b). There is a large mass, with convex lateral borders, extending into the superior mediastinum, and resulting in tracheal deviation and narrowing. Calcification may sometimes be seen within the mass. These goitres are rarely associated with thyrotoxicosis or a malignant tumour, and generally occur in women over the age of 40.

Mediastinal masses tend to occur in predictable situations best seen on a lateral chest X-ray (Fig. 3.3c). In the anterior mediastinum:

1. Retrosternal goitre (5% of primary mediastinal tumours).
2. Thymic tumour or cyst (20%); aneurysm of the ascending aorta.
3. Dermoid cyst (9%).
4. Pericardial cyst or fat pad; Morgagni hernia.

In the middle mediastinum:

5. Bronchogenic carcinoma; hilar gland enlargement; bronchogenic cysts (5%).

In the posterior mediastinum:

6. Neurogenic tumours (20%); paravertebral masses.
7. Dilated oesophagus; enteric cysts (5%); aortic aneurysm.
8. Hiatus hernia; Bochdalek hernia.

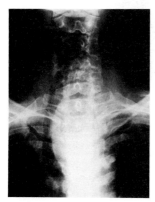

Fig. 3.3a
Goitre: close-up

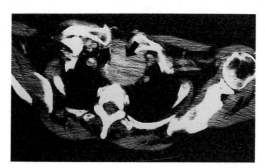

Fig. 3.3b
Enhanced CT scan: retrosternal goitre (arrowed)

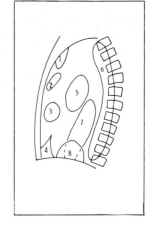

Fig. 3.3c
Typical sites of mediastinal masses: for key, see text

3.4

a. Renal artery stenosis: there is a stenosed area one centimetre from its origin.
In addition, the kidney is small, and shows evidence of focal atrophy.
b.   (i)   Decrease in renal size. Asymmetry of renal length of more than 1.5 cm
is uncommon in normal individuals.
(ii) Delay in the appearance of the nephrogram and pyelogram, due to a
reduced glomerular filtration rate.
(iii) Increased concentration of contrast medium, and reduction in the size
of the collecting system, due to increased tubular resorption of water.
(iv) Ureteric notching, due to the development of collateral vessels.
(v)   Focal atrophy in segmental lesions.

Renal artery obstruction is found in 6% of cases of hypertension. This may
be due to atheromatous lesions, as in this case, which tend to occur near
the origin of the renal artery from the aorta. This type of renovascular
hypertension is found in middle-aged or elderly males. In contrast, lesions
of fibromuscular hyperplasia tend to involve the distal two-thirds of the
renal arteries and their branches, and affect young women. Trauma to, or
pressure on the renal arteries (tumour, aneurysm) may also cause hypertension.

3.5

Acute extradural haematoma.

There is a biconvex mass of increased attenuation in the right parietal
region, with compression of the body of the right lateral ventricle. The
haematoma has stripped the dura off the inner table of the skull. Classically
these follow a temporal fossa fracture, with subsequent bleeding from the
middle meningeal artery.

In an acute subdural haematoma, blood spreads over the surface of the
cerebral hemispheres, resulting in a concavoconvex area of increased attenuation. Subdural collections are usually of higher attenuation than
normal brain tissue for the first 2 weeks (Fig. 3.5a), then become isodense,
and after 3 or 4 weeks have a lower attenuation.

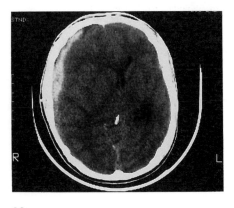

Fig. 3.5a
Subdural haematoma: hyperdense
collection over right parietal
region, with compression of the
body of the right lateral ventricle

3.6

a. *Fusiform dilatation of the ascending aorta, with linear calcification in its walls.*

b.   (i)   *Atheroma (70%): in the more elderly age group.*

     (ii)   *Cystic medial necrosis (20%): Marfan's syndrome (other radiological features include kyphosis, arachnodactyly, or scoliosis), pseudoxanthoma elasticum.*

   (iii) *Syphilitic aortitis (10%): younger patients.*

Trauma and infection (endocarditis) result in saccular rather than fusiform aneurysms. Complications include rupture, dissection (Figs 3.6a and 3.6b), aortic incompetence (from stretching of the aortic ring, or rupture of the sinus of Valsalva), thrombus formation and left ventricular failure. 10% of cases are asymptomatic, and discovered on routine X-ray.

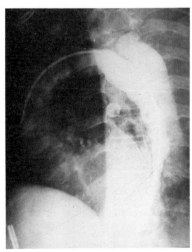

Fig. 3.6a
Dissecting aneurysm of the aorta (type 2): the catheter lies in the true lumen. Contrast outlines the false lumen

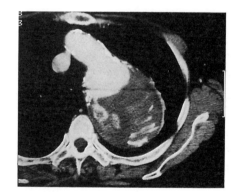

Fig. 3.6b
Enhanced CT showing a dissecting thoracic aneurysm: the true channel is opacified with contrast, and the false channel is thrombosed. Note the calcified atheromatous plaque within the lumen of the false channel

3.7

1. *Complete duplication of the left renal pelvis and ureter (duplex).*
2. *Hydronephrosis of the upper renal segment.*
3. *Dilatation of the ureter of the upper renal segment.*
4. *Ureterocele: filling defect in the bladder.*

The ureter from the upper renal segment drains into the lower of the two ureteric orifices. Ureteroceles are common. In some cases of this disorder, the ureter drains into the vagina or bladder neck.

3.8

Sarcoidosis.

Her first X-ray shows bilateral, symmetrical hilar enlargement, with normal lung fields (Grade I). One year later, the hilar enlargement is less prominent, but the lung fields are now abnormal. There is diffuse reticulonodular shadowing in both lower zones, suggesting pulmonary infiltration (Grade II). This progression is strongly suggestive of sarcoidosis.

The differential diagnosis of bilateral hilar enlargement is large. It may be due to:

1. Enlarged lymph nodes:
   a. Hodgkin's disease: usually asymmetrical, with more prominent paratracheal involvement.
   b. Sarcoidosis: usually symmetrical, with more prominent hilar than paratracheal involvement.
   c. Tuberculosis: uncommon.
   d. Metastases: usually unilateral.
   e. Rare causes: leukaemia, cystic fibrosis, specific infections in childhood (e.g. mycoplasma pneumonia).
2. Enlarged blood vessels:
   a. Left to right shunts: atrial or ventricular septal defect, patent ductus arteriosus.
   b. Pulmonary arterial hypertension (A2.13).

3.9

a. *Chondrocalcinosis.*

b. (i) *Metabolic disorders: primary hyperparathyroidism, gout, ochronosis, acromegaly, diabetes mellitus, Wilson's disease, hypothyroidism, haemochromatosis.*

 (ii) *Idiopathic chondrocalcinosis: elderly.*

 (iii) *Pyrophosphate arthropathy (pseudogout).*

Calcification may be seen in other fibrocartilaginous structures (appears as diffuse or mottled patches: symphysis pubica, annulus fibrosis, labrum of the acetabulum and glenoid cavity), and in hyaline cartilage in other joints (fine stippled line parallel to the underlying bony cortex: hip, shoulder, elbow).

3.10

Crohn's disease (regional enteritis) of the terminal ileum.

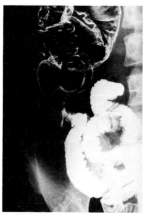

Fig. 3.10a
Ileocaecal tuberculosis

There is a long thin column of barium, with irregular margins, which outlines the narrowed lumen of part of the terminal ileum (string sign of Kantor). This affected segment is separated from other loops by its thickened wall and mesentery, which has also caused an indentation on the medial wall of the caecum.

In many instances the radiological appearances of Crohn's disease of the small bowel are characteristic and reflect the underlying pathological processes: mucosal and submucosal oedema (thickened mucosal folds), congestion and oedema of the muscle layers (thickened walls), ulceration (cobblestone mucosa, 'rose-thorns'), fistulae and strictures. In others, it may be difficult to distinguish radiologically from tuberculosis of the small bowel. More usually, tuberculosis results in an irregular contracted caecum (Stierlin's sign: Fig. 3.10a), with a patulous ileocaecal valve. Radiological evidence of pulmonary tuberculosis is seen in 50% of cases. Calcified mesenteric lymph nodes may be seen in both Crohn's disease and tuberculosis.

3.11

a. Enlargement of the azygous (right paratracheal) lymph nodes.

b. Paraspinal mass (this is visible on his chest X-ray as a shadow behind the left border of the heart, below the left hilar region).

c. Tuberculosis, with azygous node enlargement and paravertebral abscess formation.

On the lateral thoracic spine X-ray (Fig. 3.11a), there is extensive destruction of the lower half of the seventh thoracic vertebral body, with involvement of the upper anterior corner of the eighth, and destruction of the intervening disc (Pott's disease, or tuberculous osteomyelitis of the spine).

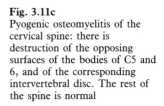

Fig. 3.11a
Tuberculous osteomyelitis of the spine

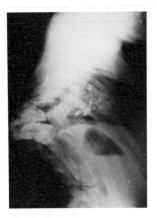

Fig. 3.11b
Gibbus in Pott's disease of the spine

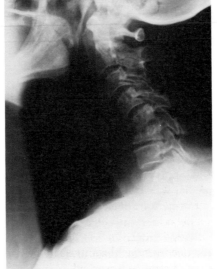

Fig. 3.11c
Pyogenic osteomyelitis of the cervical spine: there is destruction of the opposing surfaces of the bodies of C5 and 6, and of the corresponding intervertebral disc. The rest of the spine is normal

The spine is the commonest osseous site of tuberculosis, most lesions occuring in or below the mid-thoracic region. Before the advent of anti-tuberculous chemotherapy, gross destructive lesions were seen, with resultant severe kyphosis (gibbus: Fig. 3.11b), and extensive paraspinal calcification.

Pyogenic osteomyelitis may produce identical radiological changes (Fig. 3.11c). Following antibiotic therapy, the affected vertebral bodies often fuse. The radiographic picture may then simulate congenital vertebral fusion (Klippel–Feil syndrome — Fig. 3.11d), where fusion of the neural arches may also occur.

Collapsed vertebral bodies may also be due to:

1. Metastases or myeloma: disc spaces are normal; loss of pedicles may also be seen.
2. Osteoporosis or osteomalacia: adjacent vertebral bodies show a reduction in density, and the disc spaces are wider.
3. Trauma: wedge-shaped collapse.
4. Paget's disease: dense, slightly flattened and structureless body, which is wider than the adjacent vertebrae.

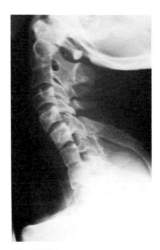

Fig. 3.11d
Klippel–Feil syndrome: fusion of the bodies and neural arches of C2 and 3

3.12

a. (i) *Sutural diastasis.*
   (ii) *Increased convolutional markings ('digital impressions', or 'copper-beaten skull'). The sella appears relatively normal.*
b. *Chronic raised intracranial pressure.*

Sutural diastasis generally implies long-standing raised intracranial pressure. Increased convolutional markings are commonly seen in normal children, particularly between the ages of 4 and 10.

In adults, radiological evidence of raised intracranial pressure is different from that seen in the child. The characteristic change is erosion of the dorsum sellae. Sutural diastasis is not seen, and increased convolutional markings are of no significance. Some causes of raised intracranial pressure, such as intracranial tumours, may also result in pineal displacement.

3.13

Ruptured popliteal (Baker's) cyst.

The arthrogram shows seepage of contrast medium between the tissue planes of the thigh. In osteoarthrosis, rheumatoid disease, or following trauma, a tense synovial effusion may give rise to a swelling in the posterior aspect of the knee (popliteal cyst — Fig. 3.13a). Such cysts may rupture during normal exercise, usually into the fascial planes of the calf rather than the thigh, resulting in clinical features almost indistinguishable from those of a deep venous thrombosis. The rupture seals spontaneously, and the fluid in the tissues is absorbed.

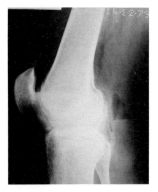

Fig. 3.13a
Popliteal cyst

3.14

a. (i) *The calyces and pelvis of the left kidney are compressed, and displaced upwards, suggesting gross enlargement of the lower part of the kidney by a cyst or tumour.*

(ii) *No soft tissue mass is seen, but there is a marked scoliosis concave to the side of the abnormal pyelogram.*

b. (i) *Renal cell carcinoma (Grawitz tumour, hypernephroma).*

(ii) *Nephroblastoma (Wilms' tumour).*

There are three renal tumours which may cause hypertension, usually through excess renin production, though renal artery stenosis is implicated in some cases. The first, renal cell carcinoma, is rare before puberty (though was the diagnosis in this case). 10% of cases show calcification. The second, nephroblastoma, is rare after the first decade, and does not calcify. Finally, juxtaglomerular cell tumours may cause hypertension, but are usually very small.

Downward displacement of the calyces and pelvis would suggest either a renal or suprarenal mass, such as a neuroblastoma which may show speckled calcification (30% of cases).

3.15

a. Large left atrium.
b. Mitral valve calcification.

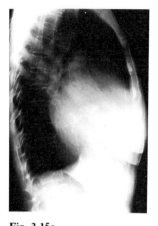

Fig. 3.15a
Calcified mitral valve

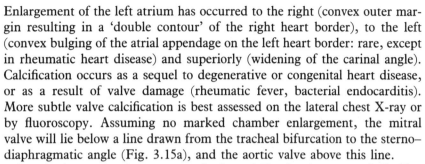

Enlargement of the left atrium has occurred to the right (convex outer margin resulting in a 'double contour' of the right heart border), to the left (convex bulging of the atrial appendage on the left heart border: rare, except in rheumatic heart disease) and superiorly (widening of the carinal angle). Calcification occurs as a sequel to degenerative or congenital heart disease, or as a result of valve damage (rheumatic fever, bacterial endocarditis). More subtle valve calcification is best assessed on the lateral chest X-ray or by fluoroscopy. Assuming no marked chamber enlargement, the mitral valve will lie below a line drawn from the tracheal bifurcation to the sterno-diaphragmatic angle (Fig. 3.15a), and the aortic valve above this line.

In mitral stenosis, the presence of valve calcification is a contra-indication to valvotomy. Two main groups of valve replacements are available:

1. Prosthetic valves: Starr–Edwards ball-in-cage (Fig. 3.15b), or Bjork–Shiley tilting disc valve (Fig. 3.15c).
2. Biological valves: homografts (cadaveric) or heterografts (pig mitral valve), usually mounted on a metal frame (Fig. 3.15d).

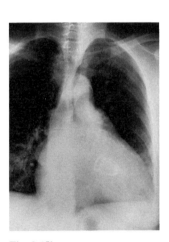

Fig. 3.15b
Starr–Edwards mitral valve
prosthesis

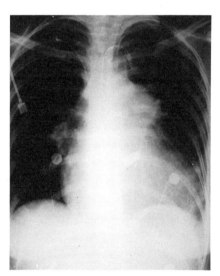

Fig. 3.15c
Bjork–Shiley aortic valve
prosthesis

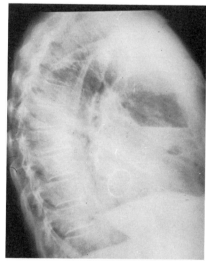

Fig. 3.15d
Hancock (heterograft) mitral
valve prosthesis

3.16

Previous chicken pox pneumonia.

There are numerous, discrete, 1–3 mm, rounded, calcified nodules evenly scattered throughout the lung fields (FIg. 3.16a). Other causes of widespread calcified intrapulmonary nodules include:

1. Healing or healed pulmonary tuberculosis: nodules are usually more opaque, irregular in shape and size, with a tendency to aggregate in clusters and in one area (especially the apices).
2. Healed histoplasmosis: virtually unknown in Europe. May be indistinguishable from previous chicken pox pneumonia. Occasionally some nodules have a dense central calcified core, surrounded by a halo of decrased opacity.
3. Ossific nodules in chronic pulmonary venous hypertension (e.g. mitral stenosis): usually denser, more irregular nodules, 3–8 mm, and in greater numbers in the lower zones. The cardiac shadow may also be abnormal.
4. Rare manifestations of pulmonary secondaries from an osteogenic sarcoma: usually in the lower zones.
5. Microlithiasis alveolarum: dense, sand-like opacities, which result in an almost uniform white appearance to the lower zones.

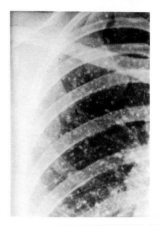

Fig. 3.16a
Chicken pox pneumonia

3.17

a. (i) *Punched-out defects in the necks of some of the phalanges ('pseudocysts': granulomata). There is no periosteal reaction, or surrounding decalcification. The joint spaces are intact, and there is no periarticular osteoporosis.*
   (ii) *Absorption of some of the tufts of the distal phalanges, and of the head and shaft of the proximal phalanx of the third toe of the left foot (neuropathic type of lesion — A2.3).*
   (iii) *Coarsened trabeculation of some phalanges ('lattice appearance').*
b. *Bone sarcoid.*

This is rare, affecting less than 5% of cases with intrathoracic sarcoidosis. It is usually associated with extensive skin lesions, and may be symptomless or extremely painful. Other sites of involvement may include the feet, facial bones (nasal bone destruction), skull and vertebral column. Other radiological features include periarticular calcinosis (hypercalcaemia in 20–45% of cases), circumscribed destructive lesions in the long bones (pseudocysts), and localized or generalized sclerosis (rare). All types of sarcoid are more common among the negro races.

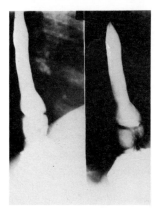

Fig. 3.18a
Schatzki's ring

3.18

Para-oesophageal ('rolling') hiatus hernia.

This is less common than the 'sliding' hiatus hernia, where the cardio-oesophageal junction slides upwards into the thorax. In some patients this junction is visible (Schatzki's ring — Fig. 3.18a), as a thin ring above the hiatus hernia with a narrow central lumen. This ring is composed of connective tissue and hypertrophied muscularis mucosa, with no contribution from the submucosa or major muscle coat, and no evidence of inflammation. This is strictly a radiological diagnosis. Clinically, it results in intermittent painful dysphagia ('steak house syndrome'), when a bolus of poorly chewed food impacts on the ring. The food is either regurgitated, or, following a drink, passes through with immediate relief of symptoms.

3.19

Malignant pleural mesothelioma

There is a thick rind of tissue, in parts lobulated, encasing the right lung and spreading along the oblique fissure. A more common presentation of this tumour is as a large pleural effusion. Such tumours almost invariably occur in individuals with an occupational exposure to asbestos (e.g. dock labourers, pipe laggers). Other features of asbestos-related disease (e.g. asbestos pleural plaques, asbestosis) may also be seen in the opposite lung.

Similar CT appearances may be seen in a primary adenocarcinoma of the lung, or in metastatic spread to the pleura (e.g. from a breast adenocarcinoma). Very occasionally, tuberculous pleural disease may mimic this condition.

3.20

a. Ochronosis (alkaptonuria).
b. (i) Pains in other large joints (chondrocalcinosis — A3.9).
*   (ii) Urine darkens on standing (oxidation of homogentisic acid).*
*   (iii) Slate-blue discoloration of the ears, ear wax and over the nose.*
*   (iv) Discoloration of the skin of the axillae and groin.*

Diffuse calcification of all the discs is pathognomonic of this autosomal recessive disorder. Lack of the liver enzyme homogentisic acid oxidase results in deposition of a black pigment (a derivative of homogentisic acid) in the tissues (especially cartilage, tendons and connective tissue). Affected articular cartilages lose their elasticity, and features of secondary osteoarthrosis develop, usually during the fourth decade. The pigment is also thought to be responsible for premature atherosclerosis.

Section 4

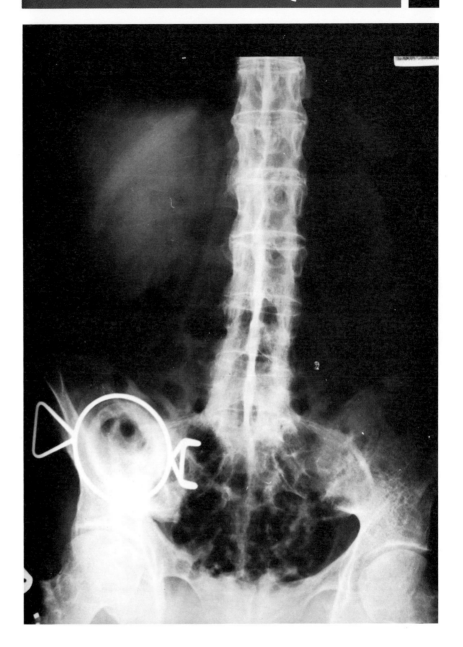

4.1

a. What two sets of abnormalities are visible on this X-ray?
b. What is the most likely cause for each abnormality?

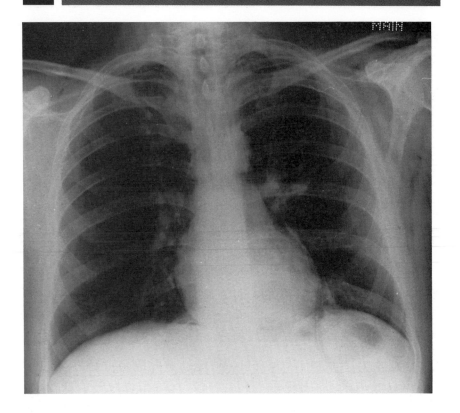

4.2

This 60-year-old man presented with severe chest pain during an episode of food poisoning.

a. What is the diagnosis?
b. What is the most likely cause for this?

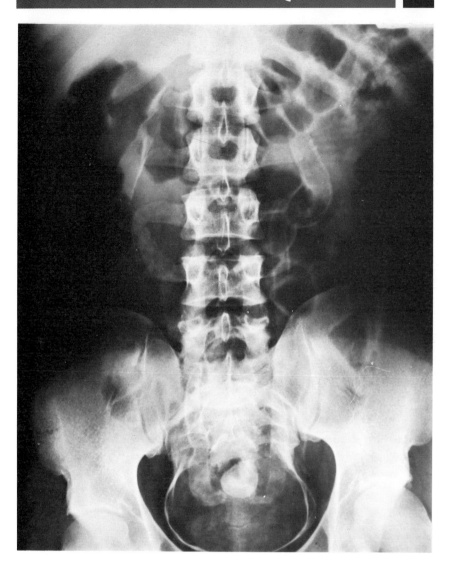

4.3

This 30-year-old Ugandan presented with haematuria.

a. What abnormality is visible?
b. What is the diagnosis?

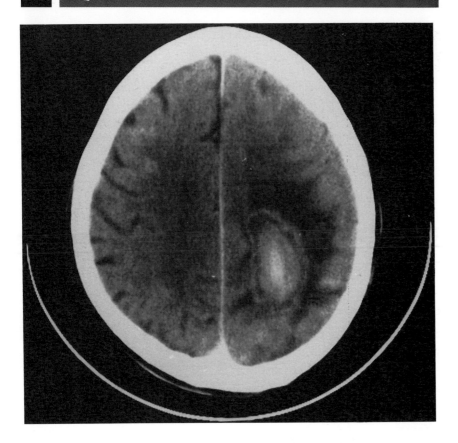

4.4

A 34-year-old homosexual man was admitted to hospital having had a generalized seizure. 6 months earlier he had had *Pneumocystis carinii* pneumonia. Clinical examination was normal.

a. *What is the most probable cause of the abnormalities visible on the enhanced CT scan?*
b. *What is the most likely reason he has developed this condition?*

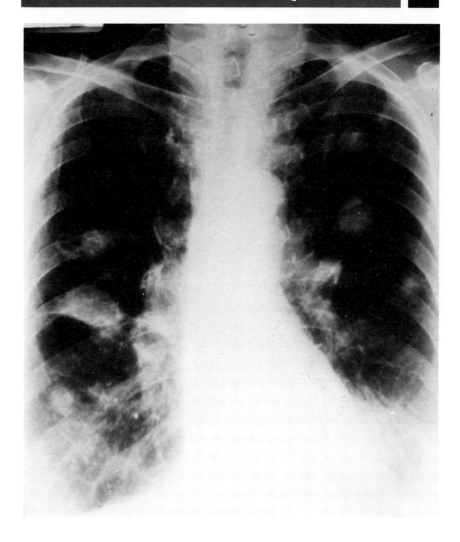

4.5

What is the most likely cause of the chest X-ray changes in this 56-year-old lady with arthralgia?

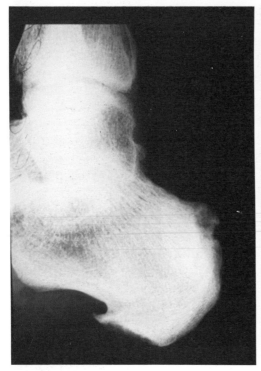 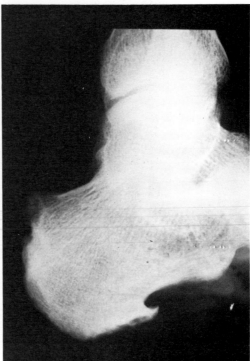

4.6

This 20-year-old man has a history of painful feet.

a. What two abnormalities are visible?
b. What is the diagnosis?

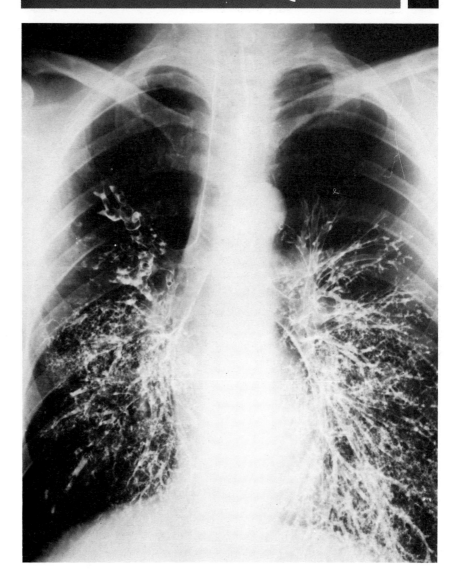

4.7

a. What abnormality is seen in this asthmatic patient's bronchogram?

b. What are the two most likely causes of this abnormality?

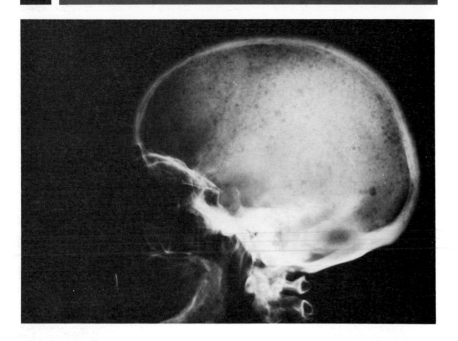

4.8

What is the diagnosis?

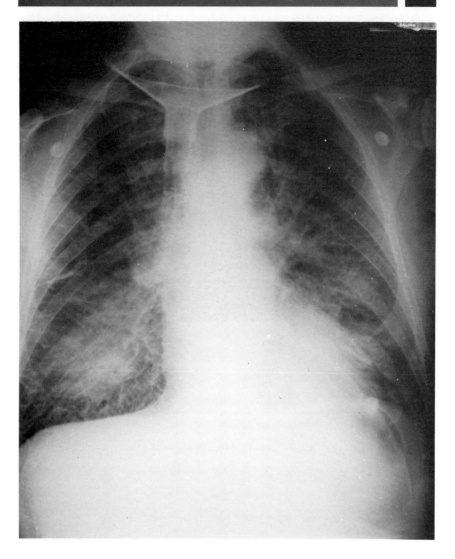

4.9
What is the diagnosis?

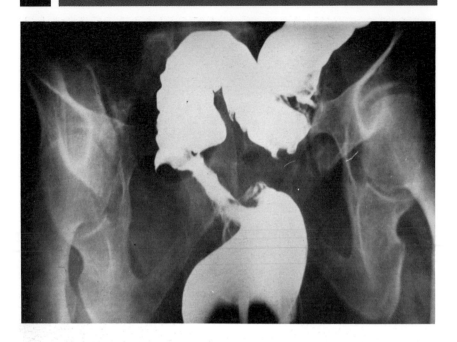

4.10

Two features are visible on this barium enema examination.

What are they due to?

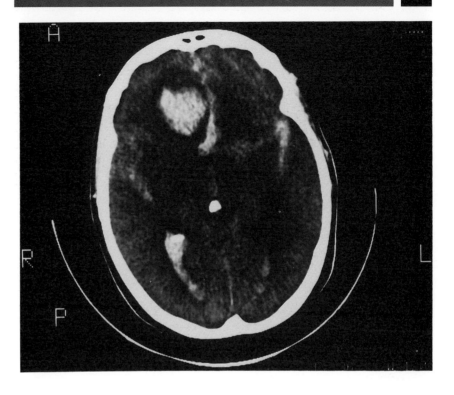

4.11

This 25-year-old lady was found unconscious at home.

What is the diagnosis?

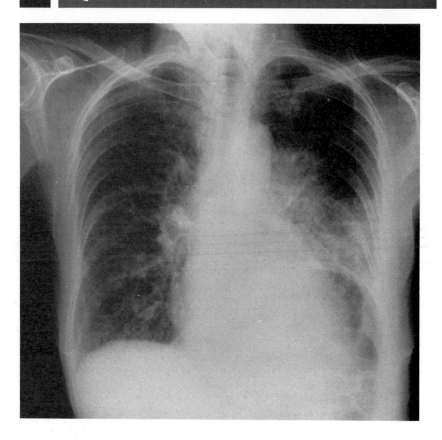

4.12

a. What two abnormalities are visible?

b. How may they be connected?

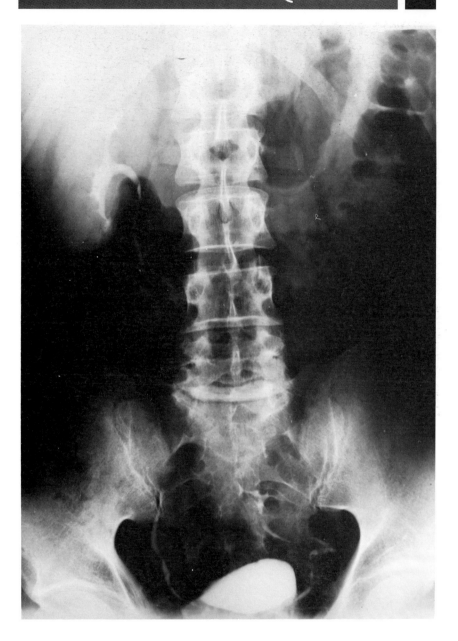

4.13
What abnormality is shown?

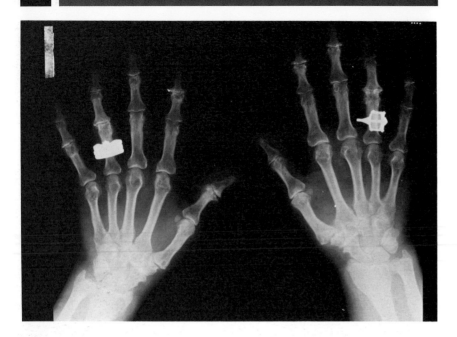

4.14
What is the diagnosis?

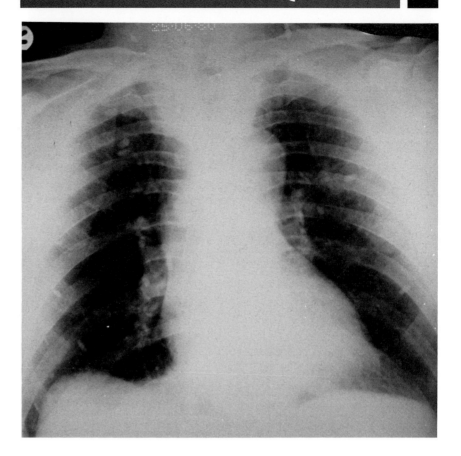

4.15

This 25-year-old Indian man presented with epilepsy.

a. What abnormality is visible?
b. What is the diagnosis?

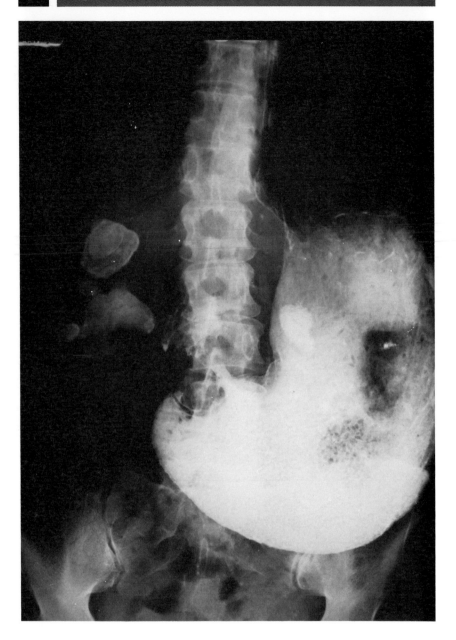

4.16

a. *Describe two abnormalities visible on this barium meal examination.*

b. *What metabolic abnormality would account for both sets of abnormalities?*

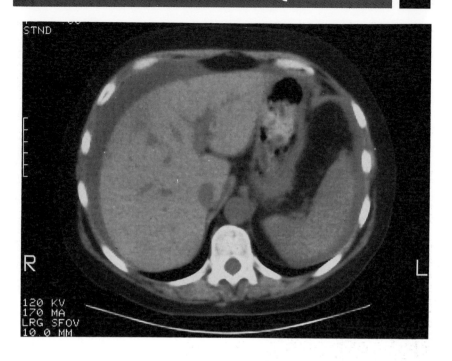

4.17

What is the cause of the abnormality visible on this CT scan?

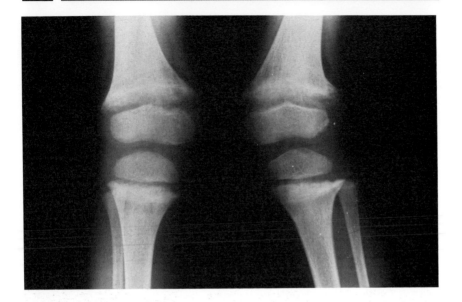

4.18

These knee X-rays are of a 5-year-old epileptic Asian boy.

a. What is the diagnosis?
b. Give three reasons why he has developed this condition.

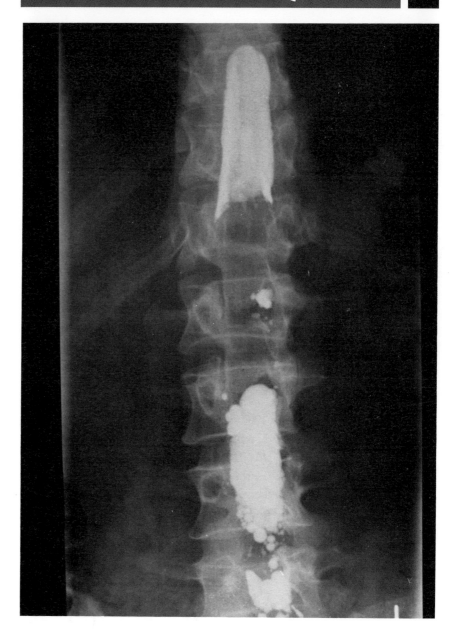

4.19

In this myelogram, contrast has been injected by lumbar and then cisternal puncture.

What is the most likely diagnosis?

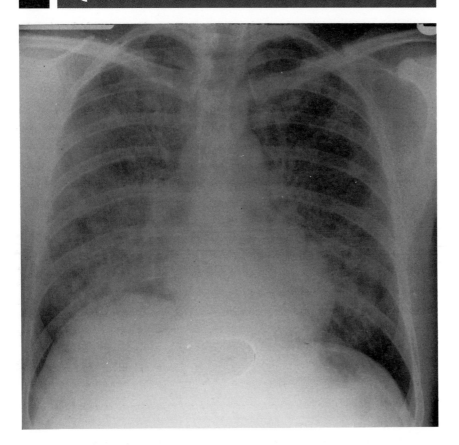

4.20

A 39-year-old homosexual presented with a 3-week history of night sweats, dry cough and increasing breathlessness. On examination he was febrile (39°C) but had no abnormal respiratory signs.

What is the most likely cause of his abnormal chest X-ray?

4.1

a. *(i)* *Bony ankylosis of both sacro-iliac joints. Vertebral body and spinous fusion, and calcification of the longitudinal ligaments ('bamboo spine').*
  (ii) *Ileostomy stoma in the right lower quadrant.*
b. *(i)* *Ankylosing spondylitis.*
  (ii) *Inflammatory bowel disease for which the patient has had a total colectomy.*

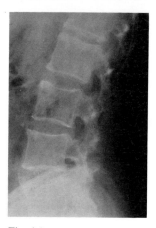

Fig. 4.1a
Early ankylosing spondylitis

There is a significant relationship between inflammatory bowel disease and ankylosing spondylitis (AS). Over 10% of patients with classical AS will be found to have ulcerative colitis or Crohn's disease. Conversely, 5% of cases of ulcerative colitis develop a seronegative arthropathy which is clinically and radiologically similar to classical AS.

Confirmation of the diagnosis of AS depends on radiography. The early features are bilateral sacro-iliitis (essential for the diagnosis); squared lumbar vertebrae (Fig. 4.1a), with filling in of the anterior concave surface and loss of the normal lordosis. Small erosions may develop in the upper and lower corners of the vertebral bodies (Romanus lesions). These changes are followed by vertical calcification in the annulus fibrosus, leading to syndesmophyte formation.

4.2

a. Mediastinal (pneumomediastinum) and subcutaneous emphysema.
b. Oesophageal rupture (Boerhaave syndrome) due to excessive vomiting.

Vertical, linear streaks of translucency outline the mediastinal tissue planes. The pleura adjacent to the left hilum is separated from the heart shadow by air, and is visible as a thin line running parallel to the mediastinum. Air has also tracked between the muscle and fascial planes of the neck. Other causes of pneumomediastinum are:

1. Perforation of the pharynx, trachea or main bronchus.
2. Pulmonary interstitial emphysema, due to rupture of an alveolar basement membrane. Air leaks into the perivascular sheaths and then into the mediastinum. This may occur in acute asthma, positive pressure ventilation, labour, whooping cough and measles.
3. With pneumothorax, pneumoperitoneum, or pre-sacral air insufflation (in the investigation of adrenal tumours).

4.3

a. Curvilinear calcification of the bladder wall and the length of both dilated and tortuous ureters. A bladder calculus is also present.

b. Advanced urinary schistosomiasis.

This disease is endemic in East and South Africa and is the result of infestation by *Schistosoma haematobium*. Ova are deposited by the female parasite in the submucosa of the lower urinary tract, resulting in an extensive granulomatous reaction, with later calcification and fibrosis. Chronic infestation may give rise to squamous cell carcinoma of the bladder.

4.4

a. Cerebral toxoplasmosis.

b. As part of his acquired immunodeficiency syndrome (AIDS): this is strongly suggested by his previous history of Pneumocystis carinii pneumonia.

There is a mass in the left occipito-parietal region with contrast ring enhancement, marked surrounding oedema, and mass effect.

Toxoplasmosis is by far the commonest cause of focal neurological abnormalities in individuals with AIDS, and occurs in up to one-third of cases. CT scanning of the brain shows single or multiple lesions with a predilection for the basal ganglia or straddling the corticomedullary junction in the frontoparietal and occipital lobes. The lesions usually show ring enhancement, mass effect and surrounding oedema. These radiological features are, however, non-specific and may be mimicked in an AIDS patient by lymphoma, metastatic Kaposi's sarcoma, and other causes of cerebral abscess (e.g. *Aspergillus*, *Nocardia* and *Candida* species).

In an immunocompetent individual the most likely cause for these CT abnormalities would be bacterial cerebral abscesses (e.g. in a case of infective endocarditis), or metastatic carcinoma (e.g. small cell carcinoma of the lung).

4.5

Rheumatoid disease of the lung, with nodule formation.

There are multiple, rounded, well-circumscribed and predominantly peripherally placed nodules. Some have cavitated. In addition, there is evidence of basal interstitial disease. These findings, together with the clinical details, suggest this diagnosis.

The commonest pulmonary complication of rheumatoid disease is pleuritis with pleural effusion (which may remain unchanged for years), and pleural thickening. Nodules only occur in seropositive individuals, and appear in crops, their numbers varying from X-ray to X-ray. Some may calcify. Caplan's syndrome refers to the association of rheumatoid nodules with coal workers' pneumoconiosis.

Other causes of multiple pulmonary nodules or homogeneous shadows (with or without cavitation) are:

1. Metastases: carcinoma, lymphoma.
2. Infections: staphylococcal, *Klebsiella*, tuberculosis, histoplasmosis, or multiple hydatid cysts.
3. Wegener's granulomatosis (Fig. 4.5a).
4. Developmental defects: e.g. multiple pulmonary arteriovenous fistulae.
5. Multiple pulmonary infarcts.
6. Progressive massive fibrosis (Fig. 4.5b).

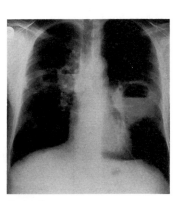

Fig. 4.5a
Wegener's granulomatosis

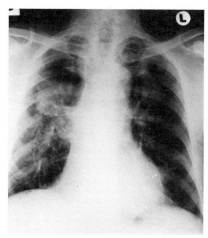

Fig. 4.5b
Progressive massive fibrosis

4.6

a.   *(i)*   *Fluffy spur on the plantar surface of each os calcis.*
     (ii)   *Fluffy periosteal reaction on the posterior surface of each os calcis.*
b.   *Reiter's syndrome.*

Periosteal new bone formation is a striking feature of this syndrome. It is characteristically fluffy, and occurs at the sites of insertion of inflamed tendon sheaths or fascia. It is best seen on the plantar spur (plantar fasciitis), and, less commonly, on the posterior aspect of the os calcis (Achilles tendinitis). Such changes only appear in long-standing disease. They must be distinguished from the clearly outlined simple plantar spurs which may be seen in other arthropathies (e.g. ankylosing spondylitis), mechanical plantar fasciitis (e.g. postman's feet), and in otherwise normal individuals.

4.7

a.   *Bronchiectasis of the right upper lobe.*
b.   *(i)*   *Allergic bronchopulmonary aspergillosis.*
     (ii)   *Previous apical tuberculosis.*

95% of cases of allergic bronchopulmonary aspergillosis occur in atopic asthmatics. The inflammatory reaction in the bronchial walls is the result of a type III hypersensitivity reaction to *Aspergillus* antigens. 70% of such patients have precipitating antibodies to *Aspergillus* in their serum. Clinically, patients may have mild asthma, constitutional symptoms (fever), eosinophilia and recurrent localized pulmonary infiltrates.

     Other causes of bronchiectasis usually show more widespread changes affecting the basal segments (Fig. 4.7a), lingula or right middle lobe:

1. Congenital: Kartagener's (with situs inversus, sinusitis) or Williams–Campbell syndrome (bronchomalacia).
2. Following bronchitis or bronchiolitis, measles, whooping cough.
3. Cystic fibrosis, congenital or acquired hypogammaglobulinaemia.
4. Lung collapse with subsequent infection:
   inhaled foreign body, inhalational pneumonia,
   bronchial obstruction (bronchogenic carcinoma),
   tuberculosis.

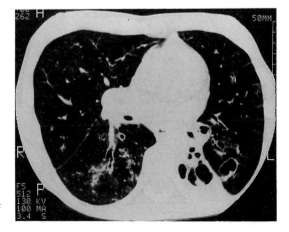

Fig. 4.7a
CT scan showing bronchiectatic
airways in both lower lobes

4.8

Multiple myeloma.

There are numerous, discrete, circular translucencies, ranging from 1–10 mm ('raindrops' — can be up to 3 cm) in the skull vault and mandible. Similar destructive foci may be found in the long bones and axial skeleton. Lytic deposits of carcinoma (Fig. 4.8a) have less well defined margins, and rarely affect the mandible.

Other causes of transradiant areas in the skull vault include:

1. Anatomical variations: e.g. Pacchionian bodies.
2. Developmental defects: e.g. meningocele.
3. Trauma: e.g. burr holes.
4. Post-radiation necrosis.
5. Infection: osteomyelitis, syphilis.
6. Direct invasion from a scalp neoplasm.
7. Others: hyperparathyroidism, Paget's disease (A2.17) and histiocytosis X.

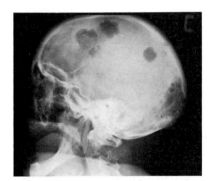

Fig. 4.8a
Lytic metastases from a breast carcinoma

4.9

Acute pulmonary oedema.

There is:

1. Pulmonary venous dilatation in the upper zones (occurs when the pulmonary venous pressure (PVP) is about 20 mm of mercury (mmHg) at rest): these vessels are usually less than 3 mm in diameter. Vascular obliteration (e.g. healed apical tuberculosis) will prevent this sign.
2. Interstitial oedema (PVP greater than 20 mmHg): accumulation of fluid in the interlobular septa (Kerley's B lines — Fig. 4.9a), peribronchial and perivascular cuffing (seen below the right hilum in this case), and clouding or haziness around the hilum. In addition, there is a fine mottling throughout the lung fields.
3. Alveolar oedema (PVP greater than 30 mmHg): a confluent shadow, with an ill-defined border, in the right lower zone. More central, bilateral fluid accumulation results in the characteristic 'bat's wing' shadow. Large pleural effusions may also be present.

The other abnormalities shown are due to an oxygen mask, and ECG lead attachments on the chest wall.

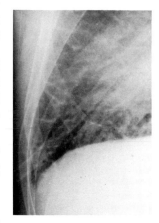

Fig. 4.9a
Kerley's B lines

4.10

1. Annular carcinoma of the rectosigmoid junction.
2. Head of the rectal catheter used to administer the contrast medium.

There is an area of irregular narrowing of the lumen, separated from normal bowel by sharp, shoulder-like margins ('apple-core'). As elsewhere in the alimentary canal, large bowel carcinomas may also occur as polypoid masses, or ulcerating lesions. The filling defect in mucus-secreting villous adenocarcinomas has a characteristic patchy appearance; in addition, some may develop speckled calcification, which may also be seen in hepatic metastases.

Rectal carcinoma is usually excluded or diagnosed by local inspection, rather than barium enema examination.

4.11

Subarachnoid haemorrhage.

There is blood (areas of high attenuation) in the right frontal lobe, falx region, both sylvian fissures and the posterior horn of both lateral ventricles. Other CT abnormalities which may be associated with subarachnoid haemorrhage include hydrocephalus and demonstration of the causative lesion (e.g. aneurysm, angioma). Extravasated blood is visible on CT in about 90% of cases during the first week after the haemorrhage.

4.12

a.   (i)   *Mass in the left hilar region.*
       (ii)   *Raised left hemi-diaphragm.*
b.   *Bronchogenic carcinoma with phrenic nerve palsy.*

Unilateral elevation of the diaphragm may occur in a number of situations.

1. Scoliosis.
2. Basal pulmonary infarction or infection.
3. Subdiaphragmatic infection or tumour.
4. Eventration: thin fibrous diaphragm, devoid of muscle fibres.
5. Phrenic nerve avulsion or crush: part of the 'collapse therapy' for tuberculosis (A1.5).
6. Lower lobe collapse.

4.13

Left pelvic kidney.

In this common congenital anomaly, the kidney has remained in its fetal position in the pelvis. It lies in front of the sacrum (Fig. 4.13a). The right side is normal.

     The commonest variety of congenital renal fusion is the horseshoe kidney (Fig. 4.13b). In this, the kidneys are united at their lower pole by a bridge of renal tissue, which crosses in front of the aorta. There is also usually an alteration in the renal axis, with the pelvis pointing posteriorly, and the lower calyces lying closer to the spine and pointing medially.

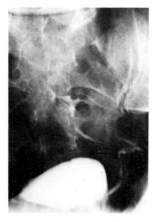

Fig. 4.13a
Pelvic kidney

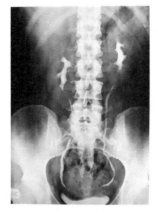

Fig. 4.13b
Horseshoe kidney: the uniting
bridge of renal tissue is not seen

4.14

Primary osteoarthrosis.

There is degenerative joint disease of the DIP and PIP joints, and the first carpometacarpal joint of each thumb. The changes visible are joint space narrowing, marginal osteophyte formation (DIP — Heberden's nodes; PIP — Bouchard's nodes) and eburnation (subchondral sclerosis). This pattern of degenerative joint involvement is characteristic of nodal multiple (primary) osteoarthrosis, which may also affect the knee (Fig. 4.14a) and acromioclavicular joints, and the apophyseal joints of the spine. Involvement of the ankle, wrist and temporomandibular joint is very unusual.

In secondary osteoarthrosis, the pattern of joint involvement is essentially that of the underlying cause (A3.20).

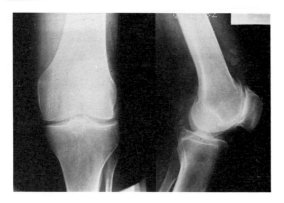

Fig. 4.14a
Osteoarthrosis of the knee: narrowed joint space, osteophyte formation, eburnation of joint surfaces, and intra-articular loose bodies

4.15

a. *There are multiple, spindle-shaped (10–15 mm long and 3–4 mm wide), calcified lesions in the soft tissues of the neck. Similar lesions are present within the extrathoracic muscles, their long axes characteristically following the muscle planes.*
b. *Cysticercosis.*

The calcified lesions are the dead cysticerci of the pork tapeworm, *Taenia solium*. Infection is usually by ingestion of infected pork, and is seen in patients from India, Africa and certain Mediterranean countries. Calcified cysticerci may be seen in any skeletal muscle (Fig. 4.15a), the heart, liver or eye. Intracranial cysticerci, a possible cause of this man's epilepsy, are found in 10% of patients with muscle involvement. In the brain, they result in round calcified lesions (1–3 mm diameter), due to calcification of the scolex rather than the whole cyst.

The differential diagnosis of soft tissue calcification was discussed in A2.14.

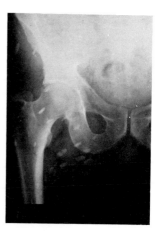

Fig. 4.15a
Cysticercosis

4.16

a. *(i)* *Staghorn calculus in the right kidney.*
   (ii) *Enlarged stomach, containing food residue; this results in numerous fill-ing defects, which in places give the barium a blotchy appearance. No barium has passed beyond the pylorus.*
b. *Hypercalcaemia.*

There are the radiological features of gastric outlet obstruction, which may be secondary to peptic ulceration (with resultant fibrosis), carcinoma of the pylorus, or adult hypertrophic pyloric stenosis. Staghorn calculus is one of the complications of hypercalcaemia, which may be associated with gastric outlet obstruction in one of three ways:

1. Patients with hypercalcaemia of any cause are more likely to develop peptic ulceration.
2. Those with hypercalcaemia secondary to primary hyperparathyroidism may have other endocrine abnormalities, such as a gastrinoma (Zollinger–Ellison syndrome; multiple endocrine adenomas type I).
3. Patients with peptic ulceration may ingest excessive amounts of alkali and milk to relieve their discomfort. This may result in hypercalcaemia (milk-alkali syndrome).

4.17

Ascites.

The liver and spleen are displaced medially from the costal margins by low-density fluid in the peritoneal cavity.

4.18

a. Rickets.

b. (i) High pyruvate content of Asian diets reduces calcium absorption from the intestine.

(ii) Pigmented skin reduces effective exposure to ultraviolet light.

(iii) Anticonvulsants (e.g. phenytoin) induce the hepatic enzymes which degrade vitamin D to less active metabolites than 1,25-dihydroxycholecalciferol.

The metaphyses are indistinct, splayed and cupped ('champagne-glass'), with an increase in the apparent width of the growth plate. The epiphyseal cortical margins are hazy. Other radiological abnormalities seen in rickets include a widespread loss of bone density, short stature, frontal bossing, thoracic kyphosis, 'rachitic rosary', lateral bowing of the legs and the changes of secondary hyperparathyroidism (A2.12).

In scurvy, the metaphyseal changes are markedly different (Fig. 4.18a). The zone of provisional calcification is dense and sharp, but on its diaphyseal side the bone shows a lucent band due to deficient ossification. This weakened zone fractures easily at its margins, resulting in 'lateral spurs' in various stages of healing. The epiphyses are small, their cortex thinned ('pencilled' outline: Wimburger's sign). Subperiosteal haemorrhages (from increased capillary fragility) cause stripping of the loosely attached periosteum, with extensive periosteal new bone formation and subsequent cortical thickening.

Except in immigrants, simple dietary rickets is rare in this country. In every case, particularly over the age of 4 years, the possibility of renal osteodystrophy or of malabsorption should be considered.

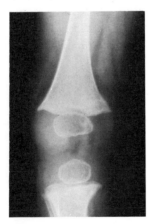

Fig. 4.18a
Scurvy

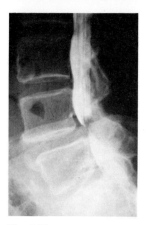

Fig. 4.19a
Posterior disc protrusion: the
column of contrast is indented at
the level of the intervertebral disc

4.19

An intramedullary tumour (e.g. glioma, ependymoma).

The concave cut-off of contrast at T12 caps the top of the expanded cord, which lies in the middle of the spinal canal. This suggests fusiform expansion of the cord within the theca, which has almost completely obstructed the flow of myodil.

Intradural, extramedullary tumours (e.g. meningioma, neurofibroma) result in displacement of the cord within the myodil column, away from the tumour whose cap is outlined by contrast.

With extramedullary lesions (meningioma; metastases; abscess; prolapsed disc — Fig. 4.19a), the theca is displaced away from the wall of the spinal canal.

4.20

Pneumocystis carinii pneumonia (PCP)

There is bilateral diffuse alveolar shadowing, beginning in the perihilar regions and spreading into a butterfly pattern with relative sparing of the lung apices and bases. These are the classical chest X-ray features of PCP, which accounts for about 90% of episodes of opportunistic lung disease associated with HIV infection (the likely underlying diagnosis in this case). This X-ray pattern is not, however, unique to PCP in AIDS patients and may be seen in bacterial, cytomegalovirus and mycobacterial pneumonias, Kaposi's sarcoma and interstitial pneumonitis.

More focal X-ray changes in a HIV-positive individual suggest (in order of frequency) bacterial pneumonia, mycobacterial infection, or PCP. The probable causes of nodular chest X-ray shadowing in this context are (in order) Kaposi's sarcoma, lymphoma, PCP, and mycobacterial disease.

Section 5

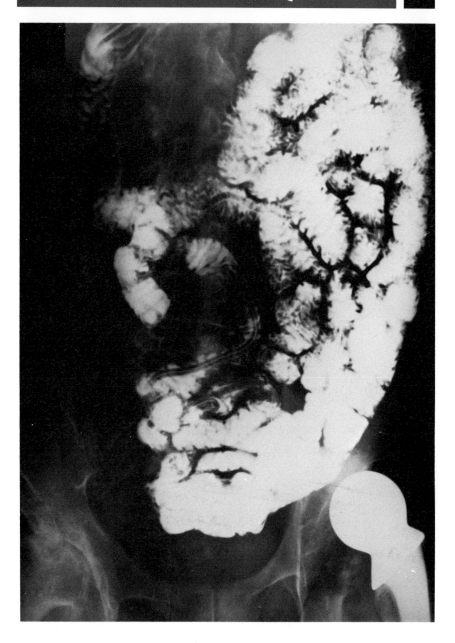

5.1

This African lady has episodic abdominal pain.

a. *What is the cause of her abnormal follow-through examination?*
b. *What other abnormal radiological feature is visible?*

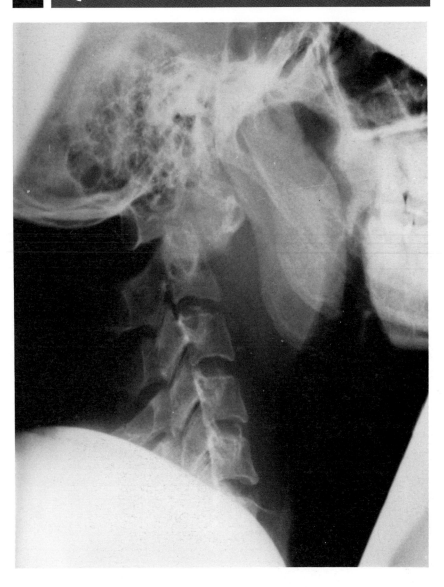

5.2

What two abnormalities are visible?

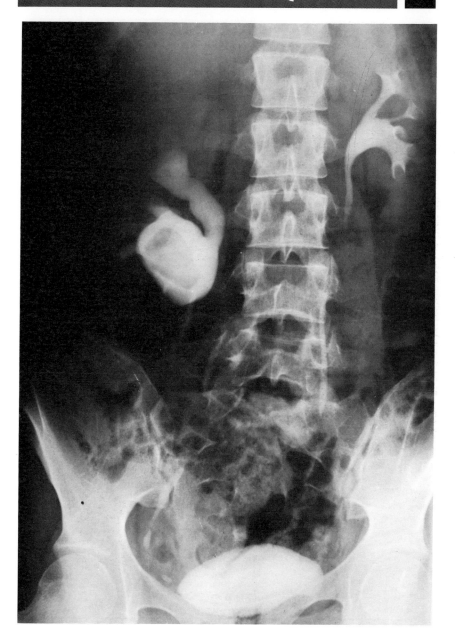

5.3

What two abnormalities are seen?

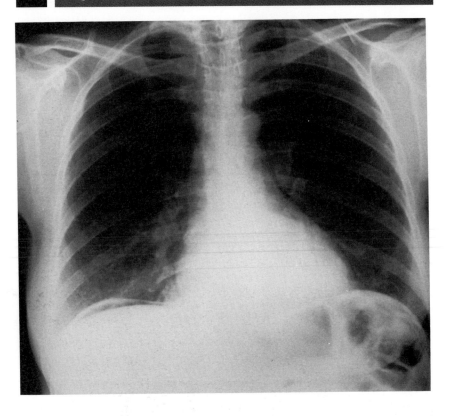

5.4

This man developed a fever 3 weeks after cholecystectomy.

What is the most probable diagnosis?

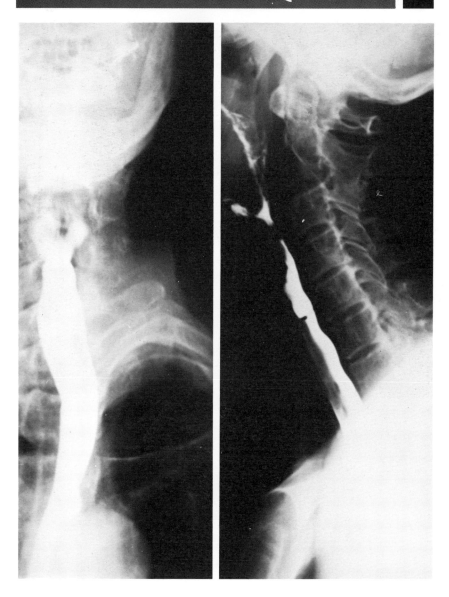

5.5

a. What is the cause of the abnormality visible on this X-ray?

b. With what is it almost invariably associated?

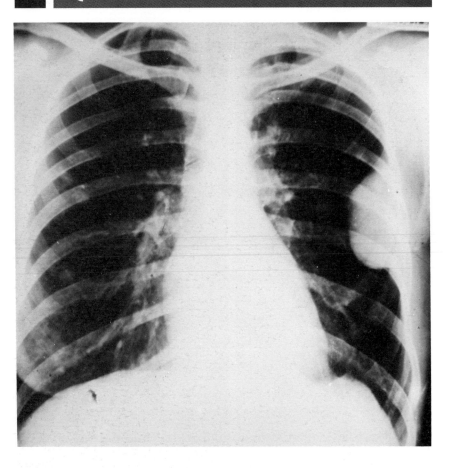

5.6

What is the most likely cause of the large mass on this lady's chest X-ray?

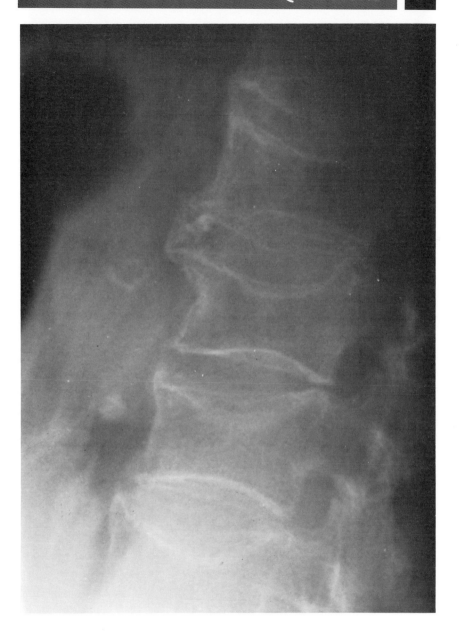

5.7

This man is being investigated for backache. Other results have shown the following: plasma calcium 2.25 mmol/l, plasma phosphate 1.3 mmol/l, and plasma alkaline phosphatase activity 160 IU/l.

a. What is the most likely diagnosis?
b. Name two other radiographic features of this disorder.

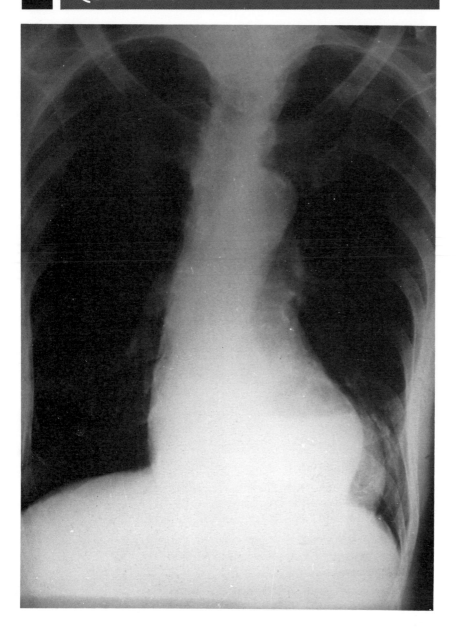

5.8

a. What abnormality is visible?
b. Suggest three possible causes.

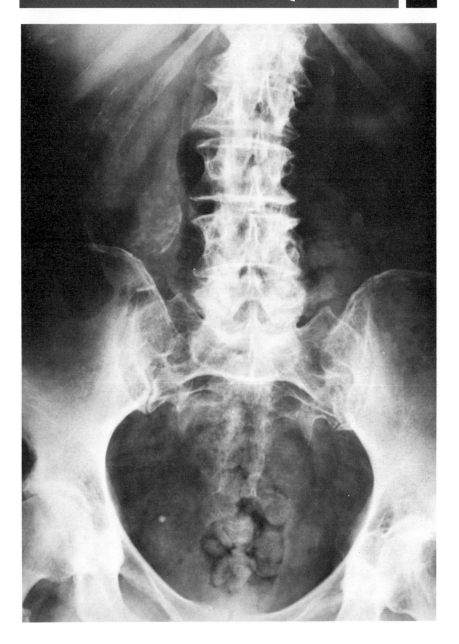

5.9

What is the cause of the abnormality visible on this X-ray?

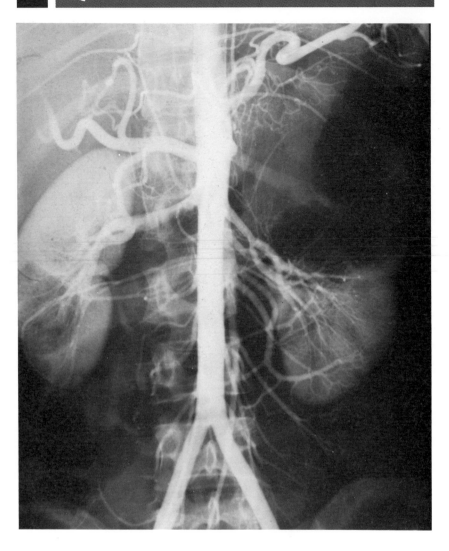

5.10

What is the cause of the abnormality visible on this arteriogram?

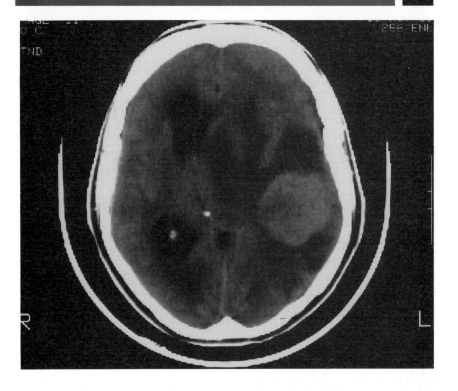

5.11

This 50-year-old man presented with generalized seizures of recent onset.

What are the two most likely causes of the abnormalities shown in his enhanced scan?

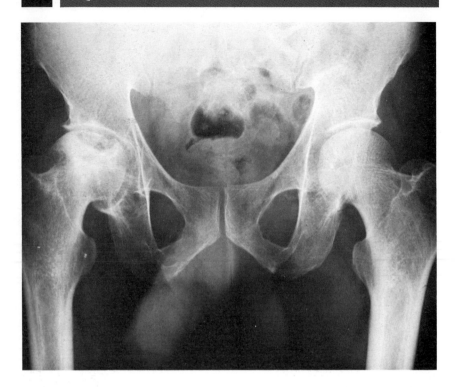

5.12

This 50-year-old West Indian man complained of pain in the hip.

a. What condition is this?
b. List six causes of this condition.

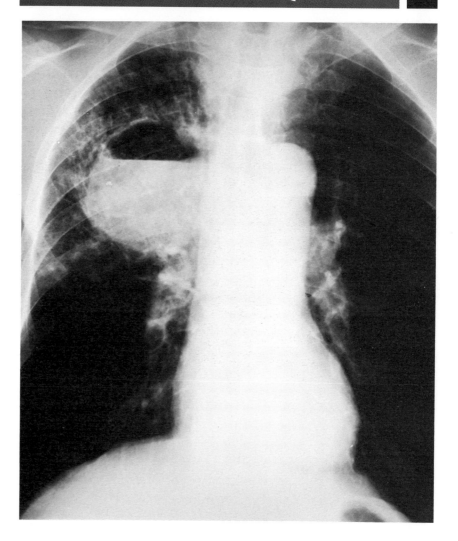

5.13

This X-ray is of a 50-year-old male alcoholic.

In order of preference, what two diagnoses would you consider?

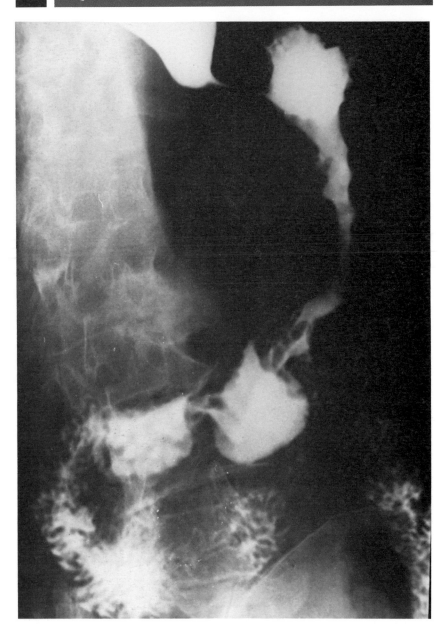

5.14

What is the most probable diagnosis?

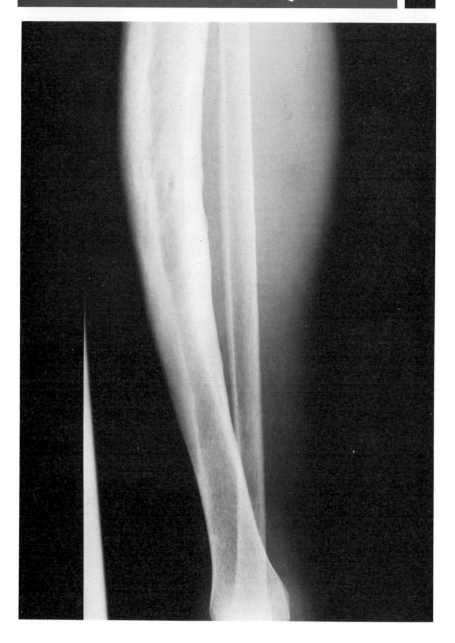

5.15

What two diagnoses would you consider in this case?

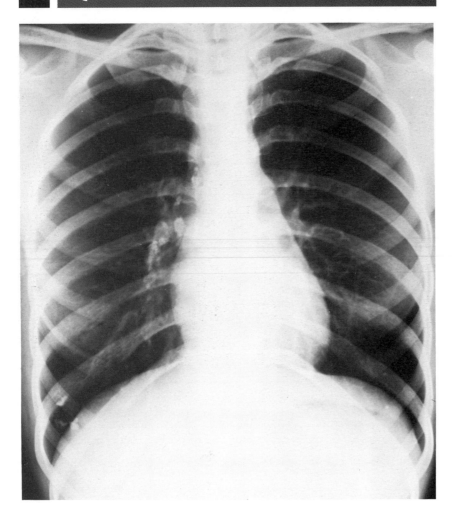

5.16

a. What two abnormalities are visible on this X-ray?

b. What is the most likely diagnosis?

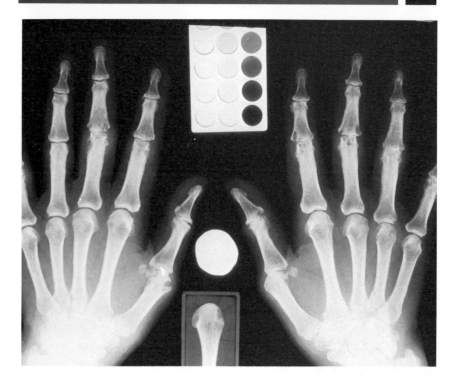

5.17

This woman gives a 3-month history of joint pain.

What is the diagnosis?

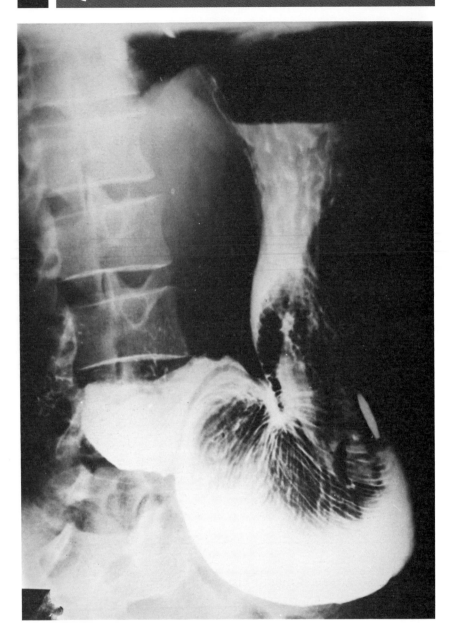

5.18

This man presented with vomiting and colicky abdominal pain. 5 years previously he had undergone an operation for 'an ulcer'.

What is the diagnosis?

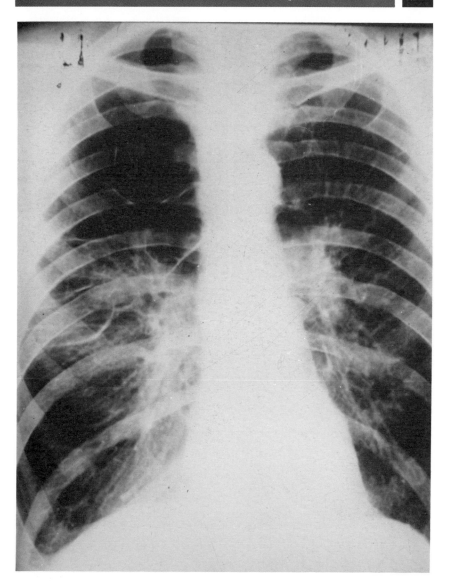

5.19

What is the diagnosis?

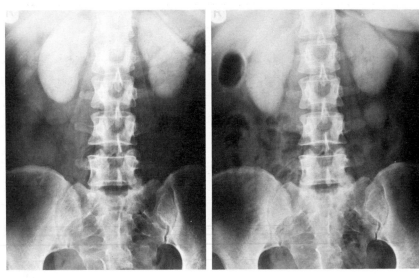

15 minutes   24 hours

5.20

What is the most probable cause of this lady's acute renal failure?

5.1

a. Ascaris lumbricoides *(roundworm) infestation in the small bowel.*

b. *The head and neck of the left femur have been replaced by a metal prosthesis (partial replacement arthroplasty).*

The body of the parasite is outlined as a negative filling defect in the barium column. This contains a centrally situated, thin, dense, string-like column of barium in its own alimentary canal. Roundworm infestation is frequent in tropical areas. In children, masses of worms can cause intestinal obstruction. Trapping of gas in between the coiled worms can give the appearance on the plain abdominal X-ray of coils of hair ('Medusa locks').

Pulmonary symptoms (cough, dyspnoea, haemoptysis) may occur during migration of the larvae into the lungs, when the chest X-ray may show non-specific infiltrates or areas of pneumonia.

5.2

1. *Atlanto-axial subluxation.*

2. *Widened retropharyngeal soft tissues, with forward displacement of the oesophagus and trachea: the radiographic features of a retropharyngeal abscess. Gas may sometimes be seen in the abscess.*

The normal distance between the anterior margin of the odontoid peg and the arch of the atlas is 3 mm in adults. Subluxation may be the result of trauma, or a complication of rheumatoid disease.

A retropharyngeal abscess may arise in a number of ways:

1. Spread of infection from a tonsillar or vertebral body infection.
2. Following rupture or perforation of the pharynx: e.g. instrumentation, swallowed foreign body.
3. Tuberculous infection.

5.3

1. *Pelvi-ureteric junction obstruction on the right side.*
2. *Filling defects in the pelvis of the right kidney.*

Hydronephrosis due to functional obstruction at the pelvi-ureteric junction is a common anomaly. Although congenital in origin, this condition may not manifest itself until adult life, presenting with loin pain, urinary infection or stone formation (the cause of the filling defects in this case — Fig. 5.3a). The disease is frequently bilateral, though usually more severe on one side than the other. Treatment is by surgery, removing the narrowed segment and forming a gusset flap (Anderson–Hines pyeloplasty).

There are a number of other causes of radiolucent filling defects in the pelvis and upper ureter:

1. Urothelial tumours.
2. Blood clot.
3. Necrotic papillae: renal papillary necrosis (Fig. 5.3b).
4. Pelvi-ureteritis cystica: a condition of unknown aetiology, characterized by numerous small round filling defects due to submucosal cysts. Commoner in young women with a history of urinary infection.
5. Air: emphysematous cystitis (diabetics — Fig. 5.3c); ureteric diversion to the skin or intestine; malignant fistula between the bowel and the urinary tract.

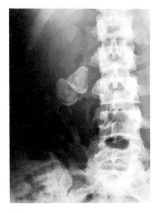

Fig. 5.3a
Control film in Q5.3

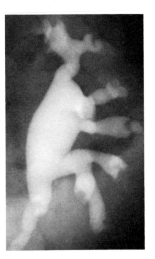

Fig. 5.3b
Renal papillary necrosis: horn-shaped projections of contrast into the medulla, cavities (sloughed papillae), and around the bases of some separated papillae

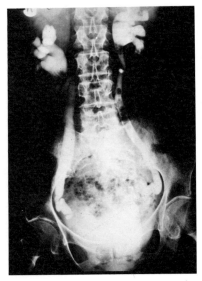

Fig. 5.3c
Emphysematous cystitis

5.4

Subphrenic abscess.

The right hemi-diaphragm is raised, and has a hazy, indistinct outline. This costophrenic angle is obliterated. Underneath is an air-fluid level. These features strongly suggest subdiaphragmatic infection (left lateral decubitis — Fig. 5.4a). The differential diagnosis includes pneumoperitoneum, which may be:

1. Iatrogenic: laparotomy (air resorbed within two weeks), peritoneal dialysis, laparoscopy.
2. Due to rupture of an intra-abdominal hollow viscus: ulcer, diverticulum.

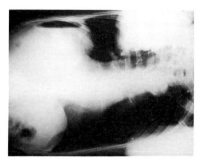

Fig. 5.4a
Subphrenic abscess: decubitus view of Q5.4

5.5

a. Post-cricoid (sideropenic, cricopharyngeal) web.
b. Iron deficiency anaemia.

The web (fibrous stricture) appears as a thin filling defect arising from the anterior wall of the oesophagus, immediately below the cricopharyngeus muscle. It may extend laterally on one or both sides. There may be more than one. Their association with iron deficiency anaemia and dysphagia in middle-aged women was first described by Patterson and Kelly-Brown in Britain, and shortly afterwards by Plummer and Vinson in the United States. There is an increased risk of both oesophageal and pharyngeal carcinoma in this disorder.

5.6

Pulmonary metastasis from a breast carcinoma.

In addition to the mass in the left mid-zone, there is no breast shadow on that side. These changes suggest that this lady has had a previous mastectomy. Other causes of increased translucency of the lung fields were discussed in A1.7. There are also several smaller nodules in the right lung field.

5.7

a. *Osteomalacia.*

b.   (i)   *Looser's zones or pseudofractures, which may progress to complete fractures.*

    (ii)   *Bowing of limb bones in advanced cases.*

    (iii)   *Changes of secondary hyperparathyroidism (A2.12).*

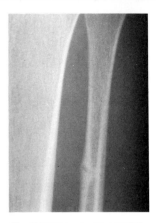

Fig. 5.7a
Looser's zone

The vertebral bodies are reduced in density and biconcave ('cod-fish' vertebrae); their intervertebral disc spaces are correspondingly large and biconvex. The epiphyseal plates are well demarcated. There is a compression fracture of L2. Identical radiological changes may be seen in osteoporosis; in this condition, however, the plasma alkaline phosphatase activity is within the normal range.

Looser's zones (Fig. 5.7a) are the radiological hallmark of osteomalacia. These 1–3 mm-wide translucencies transect the cortical margin of a bone, and represent incompletely healed stress fractures. They may occur symmetrically, in constant sites: neck and proximal shafts of the femur, ischiopubic rami, axillary borders of scapulae, lower ribs, metatarsal shafts, and certain long bones (tibiae, fibulae, humeri).

5.8

a. *There is an air-fluid level behind the cardiac shadow, together with a rounded shadow adjacent to the cardiac apex.*

b.   (i)   *Incarcerated hiatus hernia (the diagnosis in this case — Fig. 5.8a).*

    (ii)   *A dilated, obstructed oesophagus: e.g. carcinoma, achalasia.*

    (iii)   *Surgical replacement of the oesophagus by stomach.*

    (iv)   *Lower oesophageal diverticulum (A2.18).*

    (v)   *Pyogenic or malignant lung abscess in the left lower lobe.*

Achalasia may result in marked mediastinal widening (Fig. 5.8b); the absence of gas in the fundus of the stomach is a diagnostic feature in advanced cases. Identical radiographic appearances are seen in mega-oesophagus associated with Chagas' disease (American trypanosomiasis: *Trypanosoma cruzi*).

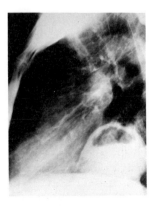

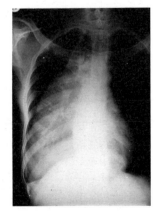

Fig. 5.8a
Lateral view of Q5.8

Fig. 5.8b
Achalasia

5.9

Calcified gall bladder wall ('porcelain gall bladder').

Calcification of the wall of the gall bladder is a rare complication of chronic cholecystitis (Fig. 5.9a). In such cases, the cystic duct is usually blocked. The risk of malignant change is relatively high in this disorder.

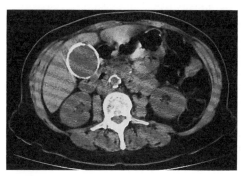

Fig. 5.9a
Enhanced CT scan: porcelain gall bladder

5.10

Benign renal cyst.

There is a rounded avascular lesion expanding the upper pole of the left kidney. Around its margin are stretched normal arteries. These are the characteristic arteriographic features of a benign renal cyst. In contrast, renal carcinomas are usually highly vascular, with tortuous and irregular pathological vessels inside the expanding lesion (Fig. 5.10a). Ultrasound and CT scanning (Fig. 5.10b) provide non-invasive methods of distinguishing these two lesions.

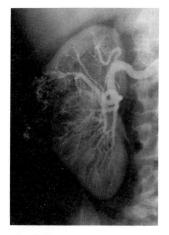

Fig. 5.10a
Renal arteriogram: renal carcinoma

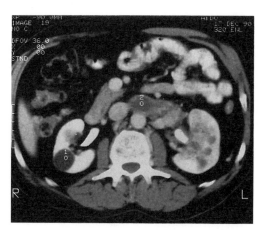

Fig. 5.10b
Enhanced CT scan: left renal carcinoma with tumour in the renal vein (cursor 2) and a benign right renal cyst (cursor 1)

169

5.11

1. Cerebral metastasis.
2. Cerebral abscess.

There is a large area of decreased attenuation (oedema), with compression of the right lateral ventricle, and displacement of the ventricular system towards the left side ('mass effect'). Within this low density area is a small, markedly enhancing tumour, highly suggestive of a secondary deposit, or cerebral abscess. Gliomas may present with these appearances, though there is usually less surrounding oedema. Distinction may be difficult, unless the metastases or abscesses are multiple. Calcification may be seen within a glioma, or tuberculoma (A2.7). In the acute stage, cerebral infarcts also show as regions of low attenuation; however, ring-shadows of enhancement are not seen. Herpes simplex encephalitis also shows a low attenuation areas, usually in the temporal lobes, and without enhancement following intravenous contrast injection.

5.12

a. Avascular (aseptic) necrosis of the right femoral head.
b.   (i)   Haematological: sickle-cell disease, haemophilia, polycythaemia, macroglobulinaemia.
*   (ii)   Traumatic: subcapital fracture.*
*   (iii)   Iatrogenic: steroids, radiation.*
*   (iv)   Collagen disorders: systemic lupus erythematosus, rheumatoid disease.*
*   (v)   Perthe's disease, congenital dislocation of the hip.*
*   (vi)   Idiopathic.*
* (vii)   Gaucher's disease; caisson disease; chronic alcoholism.*

There is collapse of the superior portion of the femoral head (weight-bearing area), with fragmentation and sclerosis. The joint space and acetabulum are normal.

5.13

(*i*) *Pyogenic abscess.*
(*ii*) *Necrosis in a malignant mass: e.g. squamous cell carcinoma of the bronchus.*

In the right upper-zone, there is a large single cavity containing a fluid level. Its wall is thin and smooth. Some consolidation extends peripherally. Its smooth, thin wall suggests that it is most probably due to infection (perhaps related to aspiration following an alcoholic binge), rather than to necrosis in a malignant tumour (characteristically this has irregular, thick walls). However, such abscesses can arise distal to bronchial obstruction by a carcinoma, and this would need to be excluded if the abscess did not respond to antibiotic therapy. Tuberculous cavities are rarely of this size, and usually in the upper zones. There are a number of other causes of lung cavities (A4.5), but few reach this size.

5.14

Carcinoma of the stomach: linitis plastica (leather-bottle stomach)

In this scirrhous type of carcinoma, extensive submucosal infiltration and fibrosis result in a narrow rigid segment in the mid-portion of the stomach. These changes should not be confused with those produced by a large pancreatic cyst, where the stomach is displaced forward, its lesser curve stretched around the cyst.

There are a number of other conditions which may rarely produce a similar appearance: syphilis, sarcoidosis, amyloid, lymphoma, post-irradiation, Crohn's disease, corrosive gastritis and metastatic infiltration, or direct extension from a pancreatic neoplasm.

5.15

1. *Paget's disease (osteitis deformans).*
2. *Syphilis (gummatous periostitis).*

The tibia shows convex bowing anteriorly, has a widened cortex and irregularly thickened trabeculae ('sabre tibia').

5.16

a. *(i)* *A group of three calcified, irregular nodules in the right lower zone.*
(ii) *Calcified areas within the right hilum.*
b. *Calcified primary tuberculous (ghon) complex.*

Calcification implies some degree of healing. Tuberculosis is the commonest cause of mediastinal calcification in Britain, but in the United States, fungal diseases (histoplasmosis, coccidioidomycosis) are a more prevalent cause. Other rarer causes of mediastinal calcification are:

1. Silicosis: in 5% of cases. Thin 'egg-shell' calcification of hilar nodes.
2. Sarcoidosis: 'pebble-like' or 'egg-shell' calcification, but no intra-pulmonary calcification.
3. Hodgkin's disease: after radiotherapy.
4. Calcified blood vessels (A1.4, A2.13).
5. Calcified mediastinal tumours (A3.3).

Extensive pleural calcification may be seen after tuberculosis (Fig. 5.16a), an empyema, or haemothorax, or in an encysted pleural effusion. Less marked calcification may occur in asbestos-related pleural plaques (Figs 2.8b, 2.8c and 5.16b), or talc workers. Discrete diaphragmatic pleural plaques may be found in otherwise normal individuals.

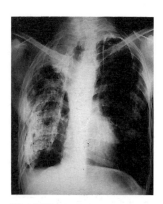

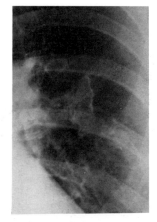

Fig. 5.16a
Healed pulmonary tuberculosis: extensive pleural calcification

Fig. 5.16b
Asbestos-related pleural plaques: 'holly-leaf' pleural calcification

5.17

Rheumatoid disease of the hands.

There is a symmetrical polyarthritis, with fusiform soft tissue swelling, periarticular osteoporosis, and joint space narrowing. In addition, there are erosive changes at the articular surfaces of some joints. The distribution of the arthritis is classical for rheumatoid disease, affecting the proximal interphalangeal (PIP) and metacarpophalangeal (MCP) joints predominantly.

Other joints which are often affected in this disorder are those between the carpal bones (Fig. 5.17a), the radiocarpal joints, the metatarsophalangeal joints, the large joints of the limbs, and the apophyseal joints of the cervical spine.

More chronic changes include subluxation at the MCP joints, with ulnar deviation; 'swan-neck' deformities (hyperextension at the PIP joint, fixed flexion deformity at the DIP joint); 'boutonnière' deformities (fixed flexion of the PIP joint, with hyperextension at the DIP joint); and bony ankylosis of the carpal bones.

Arthritis mutilans may also complicate rheumatoid disease (Fig. 5.17a) and psoriasis (A2.19). Marked bone resorption is also a feature of neuropathic arthropathy (A2.3). Gross deformity without erosive change is seen in Jaccoud's arthritis (following recurrent attacks of rheumatic fever), and occasionally in systemic lupus erythematosus (Fig. 5.17b).

Fig. 5.17a
Arthritis mutilans, in a case of rheumatoid disease: there is massive bone resorption of the ends of the metacarpals, and of the proximal and middle phalanges ('licked candy-stick' appearance), with resultant gross deformity. The now redundant soft tissue has collapsed in on itself (*main-en-lorgnette:* opera-glass hand)

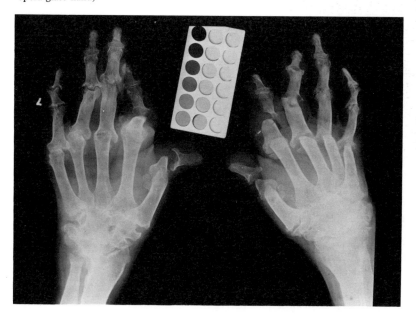

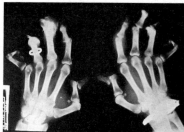

Fig. 5.17b
Systemic lupus erythematosus: flexion and ulnar deviation at the MCP joints, with marked subluxation and hyperextension of some interphalangeal joints

5.18

Retrograde jejunal intussusception.

The filling defect in the stomach has a coiled appearance, due to barium outlining the valvulae conniventes of the herniated loop of jejunum. This is a late complication of gastroenterostomy.

There are a number of causes of antegrade small bowel intussusception:

1. Polyp (Peutz–Jeghers syndrome), papilliferous carcinoma, or submucous lipoma.
2. Inverted Meckel's diverticulum.
3. Swollen Peyer's patches: infants, Schönlein–Henoch purpura.

5.19

Bullous emphysema.

There are multiple bullae: spherical or oval translucencies, with smooth almost invisible walls. In addition, there are the characteristic radiological features of emphysema (low, flat diaphragms with blunting of the costophrenic angles and a narrow vertical heart), and of pulmonary arterial hypertension (A2.13).

Bullae are seen in one-third of cases of gross, widespread emphysema. Occasionally they grow to enormous size, compressing the adjacent lung tissues and mediastinum (Fig. 5.19a). They may rupture, resulting in pneumothorax or pneumomediastinum. When the surrounding lung is inflamed they may have a small fluid level inside them. In cases of α_1-antitrypsin deficiency, the bullae have a predominantly basal distribution.

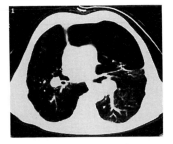

Fig. 5.19a
CT scan: bullous emphysema

5.20

Acute tubular necrosis.

Her IVU shows two immediate dense nephrograms, which persist after 24 hours. This type of nephrographic pattern in acute renal failure is seen in acute tubular necrosis, and occasionally in acute oliguric pyelonephritis.

The nephrographic features which would suggest obstruction are:

1. Delayed nephrogram, becoming increasingly dense with time (commonest).
2. An early nephrogram showing regular radiolucent spaces (negative pyelogram or 'soap bubbles': due to dilated, non-opacified calyces).
3. A homogenous early nephrogram which 24 hours later shows dilated structures.

If the early nephrogram fades after 24 hours with no sign of dilated collecting structures, there is no obstruction. Obstruction cannot be excluded if there is no nephrogram at all.

Bibliography

Armstrong P, Wilson A G, Dee P 1990 Imaging of diseases of the chest. Wolfe, London

Bartram C I, Kumar P 1981 Clinical radiology in gastroenterology. Blackwell Scientific Publications, Oxford

Du Boulay G H 1980 Principles of X-ray diagnosis of the skull, 2nd edn. Butterworth, London

Forrester D M, Nesson J W 1973 The radiology of joint disease. W B Saunders, Philadelphia

Gordon J R S, Ross F G M 1977 Diagnostic radiology in paediatrics. Butterworth

Jefferson K, Rees S 1980 Clinical cardiac radiology, 2nd edn. Butterworth, London

Resnick D 1989 Bone and joint imaging. W B Saunders, Philadelphia

Sherwood T, Davidson A J, Talner L B 1980 Uroradiology. Blackwell Scientific Publications, Oxford

Sutton D (ed) 1987 A textbook of radiology and imaging, 4th edn. Churchill Livingstone, Edinburgh

Sutton D, Jeremy W R 1990 A short textbook of clinical imaging. Springer, Berlin

Wilkins R A, Nunnerley H B (eds) 1990 Imaging of the liver, pancreas and spleen. Blackwell Scientific Publications, London

Index

(The numbers in this index are the question and answer numbers)